Mind Over Fatter

The Psychology of Weight Loss

Greg Justice, MA

Copyright © 2014 GREG JUSTICE

All rights reserved. No part of this publication may be reproduced, stored in a retrieval system, or transmitted in any form or by any means, electronic, photocopying, recording, or otherwise without prior written permission, except in the case of brief excerpts in critical reviews and articles. For permission requests, contact the author at gregjustice@aycfit.com or write to:

Greg Justice
7830 State Line Road #101
Prairie Village, KS 66208

All rights reserved.
ISBN-10: 1495247627
ISBN-13: 978-1495247620
The author disclaims responsibility for adverse effects or consequences from the misapplication or injudicious use of the information contained in this book. Mention of resources and associations does not imply an endorsement.

Cover design: Doug Coonrod

DEDICATION

To anyone who's ever struggled with their weight.

CONTENTS

	Acknowledgments	i
Chapter 1	The Diet Craze and Crazy Dieting - Our Preoccupation with Diet and Weight	1
Chapter 2	Dealing with Body Dissatisfaction	7
Chapter 3	Physical vs. Emotional Hunger - Are You Living to Eat, or Eating to Live?	15
Chapter 4	Preparing for the Journey	23
Chapter 5	Goal Setting	35
Chapter 6	Best Practices - Which Approach is Right for You?	41
Chapter 7	Strategies for Controlling Your Emotional Triggers and Stress Overeating	51
Chapter 8	Lifestyle Changes in Food and Nutrition	63
Chapter 9	Lifestyle Changes: Activities and Exercise	85
Chapter 10	Keeping It Off and Staying Healthy	97
	References	105
	About The Author	109

ACKNOWLEDGMENTS

"Rule Your Mind Or It Will Rule You."
– Horace

First and foremost, I would like to thank my family – my mother, who was my biggest fan and supporter; my father, who taught me to work hard, be disciplined and have a positive attitude; my big brother, who kept me in line when I needed a kick in the behind; and my wife and kids for their love and support throughout this incredible journey.

Mind Over Fatter: The Psychology of Weight Loss is a compilation of work from more than three decades as a fitness professional. I would like to thank all of my clients, many of who have been with me for more than 20 years, for their assistance, support, and encouragement throughout my career.

I also wish to thank my support team - Cynthia Lechan Goodman for her research and support; Nancy McDonald for layout and editing; Doug Coonrod for his book design; and Ramona McCallum for editing and proofreading.

This book has been a rewarding journey, a journey that I have enjoyed sharing with each and every one of you.

1
THE DIET CRAZE AND CRAZY DIETING
– OUR PREOCCUPATION WITH DIET AND WEIGHT

"Do I look fat in this?"

Diet, weight and weight loss are on the minds of millions of Americans. The perception of being, or even just *looking*, fatter than you want to is a national obsession. This has spurred a plethora of diets, weight loss centers and plans, regimens, supplements and has sparked a billion dollar industry. Fitness and dieting are no longer only the passion of "gym rats," but have become a heavy topic weighing on the hearts and minds of many of us!

A recent survey by The Calorie Control Council reveals that 82% of the population is either dissatisfied with their weight, wishing to reduce their weight, or are trying to control or maintain their weight. In 2010, 50% of adults - an increase from 40% in 2004 - said they needed to lose a minimum of 10 pounds.

The Stats on Being Fat

There are 100 million dieters, and 20 million of those dieters average four to five attempts each year to lose weight.

Two-thirds of the population has made a serious effort to lose weight - between one and ten times over a five-year period.

According to the National Eating Disorders Association, on any given day, 45% of women are on a diet, and more shocking than that - 40% would exchange three to five years of life to have their weight loss goals satisfied!

According to the CDC, the percentage of adults, age 20 and over who are overweight is a huge 69.2%. About 77% of them are trying to lose weight.

The weight loss industry generates 60 billion dollars a year. Devices and regimens - especially those that offer a quick easy fix for today's click and connect world - are all the rage.

Despite such timely statistics, dieting and even fad diets and unusual ideas for quick weight loss are not just recent phenomena.

It's believed by many historians that back in 1087, William the Conqueror may have invented the first fad diet. As the legend goes, since he found himself too heavy to ride his horse, he chose an all-liquid diet of liquor. But as fad diets often reveal, William's diet didn't work and he died ironically a year later from falling off his horse.

Speaking of drinking, using vinegar to cleanse and lose weight has long been a fad. For instance, in 1820, Lord Byron was reported to have drunk a great deal of vinegar and water. It's grown in popularity to drink only a combo of cider vinegar, lemon juice and cayenne pepper for a certain period of time.

The cabbage soup diet has been a fad for many years, espousing eating as much cabbage soup as one can stomach, along with a very few select foods on specific days for a seven day plan. For example, one would eat fruit the first day, raw vegetables the second - and so forth.

Today, new and old weight loss fad diets are promoted everywhere with billions of dollars spent, but they result in a relatively small percentage of weight loss success for dieters, especially long-term success. Health professionals agree that many of these fad diets can be unhealthy and even dangerous for the body. Single food or juice diets can result in lean muscle breakdowns and lowering of metabolism.

Furthermore, research has shown these types of quick losses are quickly piled back on, thus prompting a vicious cycle of fad dieting. Yo-yo dieting like this often results in having to eat less for longer periods to lose the same amount of pounds.

The Body-Brain Connection

Americans are heavier than ever and still trying to lose weight, but not all are successful. Nearly half of those who attempt to lose weight are unable to. What makes the difference between those who diet with desired outcomes and those who don't? What's more, what makes the difference between those who lose weight *and* manage to keep it off and those who can't?

In one recent year, 103 million Americans (which is 45% of adults) did lose some weight. But the frustrating part for them was that most - 2/3 of the dieters - were not able to maintain this loss, and during the next year, half of the total number of dieters tried at least two more times to diet and lose weight.

The Calorie Control Study investigated the reasons and obstacles to participants' dissatisfaction with weight loss. Participants in the study reported that they believed the following issues contributed to their inability to achieve their weight goals:

69% said not enough exercise

62% felt it was about slowing metabolism

52% believed too much snacking was a major factor

50% of women stated emotional reasons

44% of men stated their overeating at meals was a major factor

When psychological and science health professionals look at reasons and obstacles to weight goals and weight control, many agree that as a whole, Americans feel all fat is bad. We have a societal aversion to fat - especially aesthetically. But despite our visual preferences, scientific research shows there is a strong bodily instinct to store fat, and that is what makes diet and weight loss so complex.

Psychologists specializing in obesity at the Weight Wise Bariatric Program in Oklahoma City explain that the problem is that the body and brain are designed to eat, and that obesity is not just a matter of laziness or emotions, but a complex combination of biology, environment, availability of unhealthy foods, persuasive advertising, personal problems, school and fast food lunches, artificial additives, excess consumption of sugar or corn syrup, and poor eating habits. Any one or a combination of these factors presents weight challenges to us all, and preoccupation with diet and weight loss for many has escalated to an unhealthy obsession.

It is interesting to note that at one time, diet was really about food and good nutrition - people focused on the basic food groups and balanced the correct amount of vitamins and minerals from foods. Nowadays, use of diet for well being does exist - for mind, spirit, physical and emotional health, as well as for health protection - but is often overshadowed by weight loss plans and supplements, designed to lose pounds and inches rather than provide optimal well being and a healthy lifestyle.

Even the meaning of the word "diet" has changed in the minds of most Americans. Today, too many people think a "diet" is something you need to be "on" to lose weight, and not that a "proper diet" is a way of life, your surest way to health, vitality and a long life!

To succeed, most health experts agree it takes a lifestyle change - permanent changes in eating and exercise habits - to reach and maintain a healthier weight that can be maintained for life. Most will advise that it's about calories-in and calories-out, reducing calories while eating a balanced diet, and burning calories through physical activity.

Even small lifestyle changes to halt the progression of weight gain are often recommended, changes such as simply cutting 100 calories each day, increasing regular exercise, keeping an eye on and reducing portions, and recognizing and limiting fat and sugar intake.

However, as the chapters ahead describe, making and maintaining those kinds of lifestyle changes are as much about reworking your way of thinking about weight and weight loss, as they are about working out!

GREG JUSTICE

2
DEALING WITH BODY DISSATISFACTION

"Belly and Beach Disasters!" "Who's Flaunting Flat Abs?" "Thunder Thighs…"

Both ideal and unacceptable bodies are top news. They're everywhere. Even young children can't get away from being bombarded with images of bodies that the media touts as "good" or "bad," and even these tiny tykes are stressing out over whether or not they measure up!

Children are imitating their adult role models who are obsessed with the need to be slim, trim, muscled, or "modelesque" in order to succeed.

Even kids feel they must do something to change their body appearance and weight so they can be thin and "in."

Self-Assess Your Own Body Image

Consider a few sentences for a moment, to see how your own thinking revolves around food and your body.

- When you eat what you feel is a large meal and feel too full, do you think, "I'm fat?"
- When you are in a bad mood, do you usually find yourself criticizing your body?
- If something leaves you feeling stressed, do you then think negative thoughts about your body?

The Bad Fat, The Good Thin

Bad feelings about feeling fat are very common among children. A recent study by the *Journal of Youth and Adolescence* reported that a significant percentage of school aged girls wanted a thinner body, and one in four children between the young ages of 7-10 have dieted or restricted their eating to lose weight.

Children, tweens and teens base selections of friends, worry about "fitting in" and see their social skills and abilities as being related to or even hinging on the importance of having the ideal thin physical appearance.

A recent study published by the *Journal of Pediatric Psychiatry* investigated children's reactions to pictures of smaller/thinner girls, as compared to their reactions to pictures of larger/heavier girls. The study revealed that kids associated such attributes as niceness, friendliness, and kindness with thinner appearances, but heavier appearances were associated with bad, nasty, and mean characters traits. These kids also wished to be thinner and not like the fatter images.

With these findings in mind, one can understand how hospitalizations for kids under 12 with eating disorders more than doubled between 2000-2006, and cosmetic surgery rose 20% since 2008.

As far as adults go, about 80% of women are reported to be unhappy with their body's appearance and weight. This dissatisfaction is something that occupies time and energy. Body dissatisfaction can be accompanied with unreasonable amounts of time spent worrying about weight, calories, food consumption and restriction.

The National Eating Disorders Association found that on average, Americans think about their bodies eight times a day. In a recent study of college students, even 74% of normal weight woman and 46% of normal weight men thought about their body appearance and weight either "all of the time" or "frequently."

Fatness and Your Character

Thin and muscular bodies are not just "in" but signify to many people special characteristics including those of being a hard worker, successful, beautiful, popular, strong, and self-disciplined.

On the other hand, fat physiques are associated with being lazy, hated, weak, ugly, stupid, lacking will power, or a pushover.

Psychologists describe this phenomenon of thin and fat no longer being mere descriptions of appearance but signifiers of an entire moral character. Fat is bad, wrong, and dangerous, while thin is "right" and good.

Fixated With Focus and Fixing

Psychology also offers an additional explanation for peoples' unreasonable focus on the body and dissatisfaction - such focus serves as a handy distraction from other apparently too challenging struggles of life in our world today.

When people focus on their bodies, trying to change their shape or size, they receive a concrete answer to their distress. They hear plenty of supportive promotional advertising from the diet industry that assures there is an easy, simple and quick solution able to grant their wish to get slim. Solutions to complex personal problems and situations of living today don't often rest completely in one's control, so shifting focus to one's unrelated body weight, size and shape seems like a problem that's easier to understand and control when feeling out of control in other areas of life.

But psychologists caution, when people displace distress onto their bodies and try to "fix" their bodies, this can negatively impact their perceptions regarding normal relationships and distort their perspectives on activities, body image, and eating.

Another recent study with men revealed more psychological factors influencing their need to deal with a perceived unacceptable body. The study showed that watching music videos and prime time TV tended to contribute to male body dissatisfaction and lead to risky behaviors to try to "fix" their bodies.

The psychological reasoning behind this is that repeatedly seeing the same images of "perfect" bodies reinforces beliefs and values that those bodies are real and attainable, and therefore one's own "not perfect" body is unacceptable.

Unrealistic Body Image and Unhealthy Weight Loss

Many psychologists agree that the more people focus on their bodies, the more dissatisfied and worse they tend to feel about their bodies.

Statistics indicate that much body dissatisfaction today involves an unrealistic or distorted perception of size and shape. Normal weight individuals perceive themselves as not normal, and needing to change to reach their perceived ideal of themselves. And this is generally accompanied with feelings that one's size and shape mean personal failure, or negative self worth. Low self-esteem, anxiety, depression, sexual dysfunction, dieting and diet extremes and disorders, diminished mental and social performance, even dangerous practices to control weight such as exercise compulsion, laxative abuse, vomiting and steroid abuse all stem from these feelings.

A fanatical form of negative body image is termed BDD - Body Dysmorphic Disorder - in which people with the disorder are so obsessed with what they believe are flaws in their body that relationships, school, or work become problems.

Body dissatisfaction is one of surest ways to get in a vicious cycle of unhealthy weight loss, according to therapists at Green Mountain at Fox Run, a healthy living retreat in Vermont. They reveal that if the motivation to lose weight is appearance, this works against losing weight because it is accompanied by depression and anxiety - individuals feel the journey is too hard, too long, too far, and not fast enough. Instead, these therapists at Green Mountain suggest the key motivation to losing weight , rather than to look good, should be to get healthy and feel good.

From Contempt to Content

The fit and look of clothes really do contribute to anyone's kempt and attractive appearance - adding to or subtracting from your personal best. But, whether or not others advise you about clothes, make sure you dress to express yourself, and buy what you like that fits you now, not later.

Make sure clothes you wear are absolutely comfortable and that you feel good and proud in them so they help set up your mood for the day.

Cut out labels showing size, and stay away from the scale. If you need to keep track of your weight, wait for a doctor's apportionment. The numbers can cause unnecessary preoccupation and anxiety - and they don't tell you enough about your heath and body composition.

When you go to a scale, it is as if you are asking that machine, "am I okay and can I feel good about myself?" It is *always* ok to feel good about yourself. Don't let the scale tell you any differently.

Recognize and work with your genetic inheritance and see what you have, not as a limitation, but as your personal best.

Refrain from "fat talk" with friends and relatives, which reinforces dissatisfactions.

Change your self-talk about your body to the positive; don't give up even when in the beginning it can feel forced or artificial.

Before you view yourself in the mirror in the morning, set your feelings and mood with self-talk such as, "I'm awesome" and "I'm looking good," and that will be how you see your reflection. Look to see your "I'm proud of me" face.

Avoid fashion magazines and online entertainment news, which feature unrealistic, fantasy world, over-sculpted, and "photoshopped" people. Instead, pick out areas of your hobbies or interests, and flip through those types of publications.

Make an honest list of every quality you like about yourself because that is what makes you beautiful, acceptable, lovable, and ultimately satisfied.

GREG JUSTICE

3
EMOTIONAL VS. PHYSICAL HUNGER
– ARE YOU LIVING TO EAT OR EATING TO LIVE?

Recent research on obesity has uncovered some bombshell factors that contribute to the challenges and difficulties people face concerning weight gain and weight loss. It has long been believed by most of us, and even backed up by scientific research, that weight loss was mainly a matter of eating less and working out more.

However, more recent medical discoveries reveal that the way an individual's body reacts to diet and exercise has almost as much to do with **what** they eat and **how** they work out!

Why?

Because metabolism, or how your body either stores or burns fat, is all regulated by hormones. That part isn't news; science has known that for years. But the revolutionary breakthroughs in obesity treatments are coming from a greater understanding of precisely how hormones do what they do. And more importantly, how their effects are influenced by emotional, physical and environmental factors.

The New England Journal of Medicine reported on a study which supports biologists' belief that evolution has truly shaped the body to survive any type of perceived starvation with an intense and vigorous hormonal reaction. Levels of what is now know as an appetite stimulating hormone - gherlin - was measured at a significantly higher level before participants began dieting; while levels of an appetite suppressing hormone - peptide YY - were very low. Additionally, levels of leptin, the hormone that both suppresses hunger and raises metabolism, stayed lower. The study summed up its findings to report that humans have a well-organized, multi-faceted response to types of dieting. This response specifically directs the body toward putting on weight. To prevent starvation during the often-lengthy stretches between the meals of our hunter-gatherer ancestors, the body system was strongly designed to stop weight loss, and encourage weight gain.

A weight loss of 1% of body weight signifies an energy state in the body - the body slows metabolism to burn less fuel, and resets metabolism by learning to adapt to less calories. Even muscle fibers seem to change in order to become more fuel-efficient by burning up fewer calories in exercise than before. So when an individual stops this type of diet and begins to eat more, extra calories are stored as fat. This takes place after around 8 weeks of restrictive dieting and can continue for years.

It is interesting to note that in terms of overall body composition, the human body has about 10 times more fat storing cells than other cells - a ratio very similar to that of polar bears!

Other studies by Columbia University indicated that dieters would be required to eat about 400 less daily calories than normal after the diet ends to be able to maintain their weight after losing those pounds.

How You Fit Into Your Jeans May Be Predetermined By Your Genes

Current research is also focusing on the major role of physical genetics in weight gain, obesity and weight loss. Research has discovered the FTO, or "fatso gene."

Normally individuals were thought to have one, but now some are found to have two copies, and those individuals are 40% more likely to be obese than those without it.

To make the situation potentially worse for many, scientists believe there could be 100 other "fat genes" yet to be mapped, and that each person has their own number of them, with each one of those fat genes possibly able to add on pounds.

The good news is that researchers of the study believe that regular exercise could offset the risk of this type of easy weight gain.

Emotional Eating

There are emotional hurdles as well. New research at the Columbia University Medical Center indicates the brain actually changes in terms of how it reacts to food after dieting with both an increase in emotional response to food and a decrease in those mechanisms that produce restraints on eating.

Regardless of your genetic makeup, there are some sure fire signs to determine if you are primarily a physical or emotional eater.

Take a moment to consider the following:

When you're upset, do you turn to food first as a reliable support system before contacting a personal friend or close relative?

Do you eat without feeling very hungry?

Do you find yourself eating without even realizing you are eating and all of a sudden the whole dish is demolished?

These are just a few questions to begin asking yourself as you begin to distinguish physical hunger from emotional hunger - so you can know what may be contributing to your difficulties concerning weight gain, loss and stabilization.

What Distinguishes Physical Hunger?

1. Physical hunger comes on gradually and is a slow progression of physical cues such as feeling irritable, not thinking clearly, a headache, grumpiness, dizziness, lightheadedness, low energy, an emptiness or pain in the stomach. It may begin with a little rumble in the stomach that can grow into a gnawing growl that is felt throughout the body.

2. Physical hunger requires your body to eat, but does not demand specific foods. Physical hunger may bow to your food preferences but is still flexible to choices and options.

3. Physical hunger may prefer that you eat sooner but can wait for you to eat later.

4. Physical hunger occurs because your body has a need to eat after using up the nourishment and fuel from your last meal.

5. Physical hunger requires your conscious choice to eat because you recognize that you are hungry and make a decision to eat to satisfy your hunger. You can consciously and deliberately choose your food and how much you will eat.

6. Physical hunger normally stops when you are full.

7. Physical hunger is a necessary sign to eat in order to live and in that recognition there is no guilt, shame or negative feelings after you eat.

8. When you finish eating, if you wait 20-30 minutes and check how you feel, you should feel better, not bloated or sluggish.

9. Physical hunger is biological and connected to your body and blood sugar. However, sometimes because of blood sugar level instability, physical hunger may come on suddenly.

10. With physical hunger, you can make a conscious choice to stop eating.

What Distinguishes Emotional Hunger?

1. Emotional hunger comes on suddenly. You want to eat now, and must have it. You're starving - it's urgent, even desperate.

2. You crave one particular thing. It must be a specific food or type of food and a substitute is not acceptable.

3. Emotional hunger begins and is experienced in the mouth and mind. You may think of what that food tastes like, and feel the experience of eating it. Or, conversely, you are

eating and not even realizing it before the whole pizza, quart of ice cream, or box of cookies is gone.

4. Emotional hunger is about a quick fix and gratification, often following a stressful situation, painful emotions, or boredom. Often, if painful feelings are causing the emotional eating, you eat to cover up or to deaden the pain. In the opposite direction, if you feel excited about something, you could react by eating because it may be difficult for you to experience positive emotions all by themselves or to celebrate without attaching food to the occasion.

5. Emotional hunger often does not stop even when your body feels full. It is difficult for you to tell when you are full or to know when to stop.

6. Emotional eating often results, at some point after eating, in negative feelings: shame, guilt, remorse, or self-hatred.

7. If after eating you're still in a bad mood, eating did not make you feel better.

The interesting thing about the new research and its understanding of hormonal influences is that researchers have also discovered that many of the same hormones and neurotransmitters that affect mood also affect hunger! Eating when a person is depressed, or "stress-overeating," is also a way to raise the brain's "feel good" chemicals such as dopamine and serotonin. Brain mapping studies have shown that when emotional or stress-overeaters reach for the salty or sugary "comfort food" they crave, the same pleasure centers of the brain "light up" as during sex!

The good news is, now that you know the differences between emotional and physical eating, and the different biological needs each fulfills, as well as how to tell them apart, the chapters ahead will help you work *with* your body - eating to live rather than living to eat!

4
PREPARING FOR THE JOURNEY

Weight loss is a journey no matter how long the duration, location, or time of the year. And, like any journey, if you really want to get where you're going, it's best to plan ahead! Even spur of the moment travel works out best with preparations to ensure that only the best takes place and that unexpected surprises are simply great, new discoveries.

New research reveals that making a lifestyle change works best for both losing weight and keeping it off. However, all weight loss professionals agree that it's impossible to make even simple lifestyle changes without having first developed a personal plan that should involve the following:

- Increased activity
- Diet changes
- Strategies that are realistic and workable with an individual's own behaviors

A recent survey by Consumer Reports and the American Psychological Association further explains that the most essential strategy for losing weight and keeping it off must involve developing a deep understanding of the behaviors and emotions involved in the weight loss process. Components that help a plan succeed include practices of mindfulness and problem solving, keeping behavior records, goal setting, and preparing motivation.

The Best Beginnings

Let's face it, choosing to make the lifestyle changes needed for long term weight loss can seem overwhelming, even impossible. The thought of "oh, now I have to exercise every day and give up the foods I love," can be devastating for people. But negative thinking like this can end your weight loss journey before you've even pulled out of the driveway! Instead, look positively at the road ahead. Rather than focusing on how far away the finish line is, just concentrate on the idea that every expedition begins with a few easy and simple first steps. After that, it's only a matter of putting one foot in front of the other.

Self-Regulation and Choice-Fullness

The best part about your weight loss journey is that you, and only you, are in the driver's seat! You have complete control over how this journey goes.

Yes, it's the empowerment you've wanted and fought to obtain since early adolescence, or even before! And new research supports how right you were and still are to desire this empowerment. When individuals feel competent and perfectly autonomous about their own process for reaching their goals, their efforts prove successful - their behavior during the journey brings long-lasting changes and results.

The power of autonomy is about much more than being self-reliant or independent. It entails how much strength individuals feel when they know the choices on their weight loss journey are theirs alone to make. Their behavior is theirs alone to conduct. With autonomy, there are no feelings of needing to bend to or listen to outside pressure; there's no tension that comes from external influences.

Consider the familiar phrases, and the emotions they trigger in your own life: "I must, I should, I ought to," and "if I don't do ___, then I will ___." Or, "the people in my group all do yoga so I should do it too." All of these snippets of internal dialog are really external motivations that indicate too much consideration is being placed on what other people think. It's an externally-driven form of motivation that forces you to be controlled by others and probably results from guilt or shame, low self-esteem, or just an avoidance of perceived negative consequences. What is most important right now is that your motivation becomes internally directed. When motivations are authentic, you begin to realize you have a true voice about your choice. You are the one in command, the sole Captain of your own weight loss journey!

Not All Goals are Created Equal

In sports, a goal is a goal. Take soccer, for example. A point goes on the scoreboard, whether the goal is the result of a dramatic drive, or a free kick. Not so when you're creating your weight loss goals. While some might argue that any reason to lose weight is a good reason, researchers into the psychology of weight loss have found that not all weight loss goals are equal. Specifically, those people who are trying to lose weight "for themselves," for their own personal reasons, do far better with long-term weight loss, than those who are doing it for others, or because of outside influences.

The research explains that those dieting because of outside influences usually create weight loss goals based on body image motivation. A need for developing an attractive image is often due to pressure from a society that values thinness over fatness. However, goals personally satisfied by one's own autonomous motivation, with no outside control or influences, are motivated by health, social connectedness, and personal growth. When your plans and journey for weight loss come from you alone, you feel competent and effective.

The problem, according to many psychologists, is that often people who fail, choose to set out on their weight loss journey for the best reasons, yet wind up choosing the wrong reasons. They also expect to be told what to do. But studies have shown that healthy and long-term weight loss is best accomplished not only when you set the goals that are most meaningful to you, but also when you do not expect to be told exactly how to cross the finish line. That is not to say you do not need guidance or help. After all, you would not want to take a cross-country trip without a road map. But it is the idea of self-motivation, and autonomous control that leads to lifestyle changes, and long-term weight loss.

The evidence research studies have found that links self-determined motivation to bring about weight loss also shows that this works best with healthful eating and physical exercise. You may be sorry to hear it again, but eating right and exercise do need to be part of any weight loss journey. But, instead of getting hung up on the things you have to take away from your diet, think about the exciting and tasty new things you can try. And with exercise, instead of it being a chore, you are in control to pick the kinds of physical activities that are rewarding, interesting and enjoyable. Either way, eat right and exercise, but plan to do it in a way that leaves you with a sense of confidence and control in what you do.

Here are some motivational keys and inspiration to consider for your unique journey:

- Delaying and/or avoiding health problems that being overweight can cause
- Ability to join in activities you feel you would enjoy
- Feeling more energetic and optimistic about yourself
- Feeling comfortable in your own skin
- Discovering new and interesting meanings or unique and enriching experiences along the journey
- Finding new and satisfying types of rewards
- Feeling proud of the control you utilize on your journey
- Making some longed for changes in your life and lifestyle
- Finding you are setting goals and taking action, rather than just having good intentions

As Easy as 1-2-3

A new study published in the *Journal of the Academy of Nutrition and Dietetics* presented evidence that the best way to lose weight is mainly a 3-fold plan:

1. Keep a food journal. Write down in great detail all that you eat and drink, including portions, preparation methods,

toppings, condiments, and sauces. You may also note what mood you were in at each meal.

2. Avoid skipping meals.

3. Avoid frequent eating out in restaurants.

The study revealed that what really supports these three strategies is developing your sense of mindfulness - in your food selection, and when you are highly aware and attentive to what and how you are eating. To be sure, with mindfulness, your choices and responsibility for your choices are self-directed, and not influenced or pressured.

In the study, those who kept their consistent food journals lost about six more pounds than those who didn't.

The Food Journal

Journaling has been described as effective by many weight loss clinicians and counselors because doing so helps dieters make more healthy choices. Writing it all down allows you to keep track of all the little things and to see the larger picture of the overall diet quality and effects.

You might use printed booklets, or ready-made apps. For the best journaling to help you be very honest, you need to record everything you eat, which means to always be prepared by carrying your journal with you. Try to be accurate in measuring and describing portions. Be as complete as possible, including how the food is prepared.

Less Meals Does Not Mean Less Weight

You may have thought or heard that skipping meals will help you lose weight. This is one of the most frequently used means to try to lose weight and it backfires. That's because you can be lowering metabolism, training your body to hold onto fat and weight, just the way it is described in Chapter 3. Studies continue to show that skipping breakfasts can actually lower your metabolism 5%. It also tends to drive you to snack, or binge, or later on to consume even more food and calories by feeling deprived earlier. Other research has supported that people who eat breakfast are slimmer.

A recent study revealed that participants who skipped meals lost almost 8 pounds *less* than those participants who ate regular meals. The study interprets the results by explaining how skipping meals encouraged binge eating, eating fattening foods, and eating more calories than before.

Taking Control of How You Eat

You may intuitively know that eating out less can lead to more weight loss. Of course that goes without saying for much of traditional fast food. But, that is not the basis of the new research. It wasn't only about the kinds of foods one tends to eat at restaurants, but the lack of control of portion size, and the more mindful experience that comes from preparing your own food that led the authors of the study to put dining out less as "Number 2" in their 1-2-3 Plan.

Participants who had lunch out once a week or more lost about five pounds *less* than those individuals who did not eat out so often. When you are eating out, you do not have control over how the dish is prepared, the ingredients, the portion size - so this takes the awareness and total control away from you.

Knowing Yourself

It may be very easy for you to spout out any number of faults you think you have. "I'm fat," "I'm ugly," "I'm unmotivated…" Now let's start checking into what is REALLY true about you. In preparation for goal-setting, psychologists recommend knowing your personality as best you can. Know what you are good at and where your weaknesses are, so that you can prepare ahead of time how to avoid your downfalls. This way it is a lot easier to plan for your obstacles and prepare for rewards. However, what is most important about knowing yourself is that it is the best way to come to believe in your capabilities, which is often one of most people's greatest hurdles.

The Road of Good Intentions

New research has shown that there is a difference between your good intentions, and your actual decisions. Asian philosophy often repeats the phrase, "there is only do, not try." The published report in *Psychology of Sport and Exercise* indicated that feelings, self talk, statements about intentions such as "I intend to exercise, I plan to go to the gym" do not consider the amount and actual effort, the actual resolve that will be put into the activity. This means you have to consider the time amounts needed, the suitable locations, any other arrangements you have to make, and the possible before or after effects on your own body.

The authors of the study explain that people think they know a true self and believe if you say you plan to do something, it is as good as doing it. But, as backed up by the study, the truth is, it often does not.

Pay Attention to Types of Foods

Physical activity and diet are important aspects of your weight loss planning. And both need to be done properly. A study done by the Harvard School of Public Health has offered evidence that there are definitely good foods and bad foods.

Choosing to eat more good foods and fewer bad foods is even an better method of losing weight than being active and eating what you want. This goes even for eating in moderation, which still does not consider the quality of what you eat.

In the study, participants were found to gain about a pound a year or 20 pounds in 20 years. Those that gained the most weight were found to eat more French fries (a weight gain of over three pounds in a four-year period), potato chips, sugary beverages, processed meat and red meat, potatoes, sweets and desserts, refined grain, fried food, and butter.

The foods that were consumed more by those that lost weight or did not gain weight were: fruits, vegetables and whole grains. Those who lost weight ate about three servings of vegetables a day more than those who gained. Dairy and fat was found not to have any particular effect.

Of note is that yogurt was the food with the highest link to weight loss. Those individuals who ate more yogurt lost nearly a pound every four years!

Your Plan of Action Begins with Checking Out Your Options

What is great for the gander may not be so good for the goose, and that goes for you vs. everyone else in the world. Figure out your schedule and what eating and exercise plan will realistically work for you. Give yourself time to get rid of junk in your kitchen and pantry. Check out health websites and alternative health recipes. Make sure you have measuring items for having a better handle on your portions - just until you see just what portions mean.

Plan for workout buddies and friends and relatives that are supportive rather than those who tear you down.

Check out local restaurants for those that provide healthy alternatives for all styles of eating.

Good Self Talk

What you say to yourself becomes your belief system, especially the more you say it. So drop the negative self-talk and substitute the positive. The more you say it, the more real and concrete your affirmations become.

Here are some suggested ways for preparing your revised self-talk:

"Even though my parents are both overweight, I know I can make my own destiny."

"Once I finish exercising, I feel stronger, renewed energy, and control of myself."

"I want to eat nutritious food that my body deserves, and I deserve."

"I made a good healthy habit today and I feel proud of it."

Mental health therapists have described this means of making your weight loss journey the experience you really want because of *skill power*, not will power.

Preparing for Support On Your Journey

Studies show that positive support adds to your success in your own weight loss journey.

Prepare your support network by involving people who will applaud you as you strive for your goals. Get together with people who shop nutritionally, or who exercise along with you.

Tell friends and family how you'd like them to support you and let them know what they might do or say that is helpful to you. Ask them for praise on your behavior changes, not just weight changes. Begin sharing healthful activities other than eating rituals - activities like going to plays, museums, and sports.

So, take ownership of your preparation for your journey. Make it your own. It's your own life. And always remember the immortal words of Yogi Berra, "If you don't know where you are going, you'll wind up someplace else!"

GREG JUSTICE

5
GOAL SETTING

Remember, you are the most important person involved in this journey. Not only are you in the driver's seat, you're also your own best goalkeeper. As goalie for your weight loss desires, your direction, strategy, development, and your play by plays are all within your incredibly individualized, specialized power.

Recently, *American Psychologist* published a story revealing that a specific type of goal setting is effective in helping participants focus their attention on behavioral changes. Termed, "task motivation," this is a valuable self-regulation process in which the person is learning about his or her performance. Revisions can then be made as an interactive process. This process of setting and achieving incremental goals can be very effective in seeing results and making on-going behavioral changes.

In other words, you'll have short-term and long-terms goals to consider. But your focus will be mainly on your short-term goals, which are usually less than six months. Your short-term goals will effectively help you work upwards to reaching your long-term goals.

S.M.A.R.T. Goals

Professionals in both health and life skills suggest that the best goals are wise, as in *smart*. Design your own goals the

SMART way - make sure they are **S**pecific, **M**easured, **A**ttainable, **R**ealistic, and **T**imely.

Specific goals do more than just generalize about a good idea. A specific goal focuses on a certain behavior. For example, "walk more" is okay, but too general. "Walk five to seven miles a day" is specific, although probably not immediately attainable. "Walk 1/4 mile-1/3 mile a day, four to five days a week," or "Eat three to five servings of fruits and vegetables, four to six days a week," might be realistically right for you, right now.

Specific goals have better results than vaguely described goals such as, "I'll do my best," "I'll exercise more," and "I'll eat healthier foods." However, when it comes to weight loss, it's wise to recognize that "specific" goals can be broadly defined. Recent studies have found that setting goal *ranges* rather than very narrow, rigid goals were more likely to have better success. By aiming for a range, you have a goal that is clear, challenging, and at the same time, it's vitally flexible.

Monitoring Your Progress

Measuring involves your observations and recordings to help you determine how you are doing with your goals. Use your behavior journals, food diaries, and exercise logs to document "How much? / How often?" This is a good way to see your own progress and get to authentically know yourself, more and more. You will notice trends or peaks and valleys, and see how you respond to circumstances, events, changes, etc. For example, whether or not TV watching, weather, and treats at the office affect your goals and exactly how they might do so.

Attainable goals are possible, although they will be and should be challenging. Recent interesting research found that overweight individuals trying to lose weight who had goals that were greater than a recommended 5%-10% of their weight indicated a stronger motivation to lose the weight. The study indicated that higher weight loss goals were not associated with dissatisfaction, but with striving for *more* weight loss, *more* effort directed at their attempt, and, *more* short-term weight loss.

One explanation given for this occurrence is that when there are several goals a person is working towards, the goal that seems realistic but easier, may not receive as much effort and attention as another goal that seems to need to get more effort spent on it.

So, evaluate your goals to be challenging enough for you. You don't have to climb that mountaintop, but don't settle for the molehill either.

Relevant goals are those that are truly important to you. Your goals are your own personal journey.

Each one of your goals can be tracked with attainable and relevant milestones along the way. Short-term goals will lead up to your long-term goal.

When laying out your journey's goals, consider your health concerns, your time constraints, and where and when things will take place. You need to account for life events that can throw you off course. Adjust for work, school, and family challenges that could present roadblocks to your success. Be ready to deal with inevitable parties and celebrations. That doesn't mean you have to give up being sociable to hit your weight loss goals, just be prepared to readjust situations to stay connected to your journey.

By giving yourself a certain time frame for reaching your goals you can track your progress and revise your goals and strategy if you need to.

Your Path Can Be Bordered with Roses…

What is wonderful is the path you create for your goals. Remember about smelling the roses along the way? You want to know that you are finding fulfillment and learning about new ways of enjoyment every day. In fact, noticing even small changes as you move along will give you a sweet sense of pride and satisfaction.

…and Some Thorns

Setbacks and failures are normal part of life. That's right, you would not be human if you had none. So plan for "if-then" scenarios in advance. Think of any roadblocks or obstacles you might encounter, and then have plans for what you will do and how you will respond.

The Impossible Dream No More

So many individuals make vows such as, "I'm never going to eat cookies again," or "I must lose 145 pounds this week," and vows like these obviously would require super humans to accomplish. Goals need to be realistic. Health professionals often refer to vows such as these as the Imperative Syndrome or the Mount Everest Syndrome. Imperatives use words like *never, always, must, every* - words that go together with frustration, rigid standards, perfection, failure, defeat and disappointment.

Realistic goal setters look to averages and are not rigid and demanding. You would probably not be very realistic to decide, "I'll only eat 1,000 calories a day every day." It's more realistic to say "This week I'll average 1,500 calories a day." Not S.M.A.R.T. to say, "I will never eat pizza again." Smarter to envision, "I can limit my pizza eating to one to two slices every two to four weeks." Instead of "I will bake pies for the group but I won't even taste anything," consider saying, "I can buy pieces for the group at that discount bakery on my way home and drop them off right away for the group at their meeting place."

In your monitoring, take into consideration those times you might take a step backwards or sidestep and include when and why it happened, any person involved and your behaviors in relation to it. This will be useful information to help you in all areas to come.

The Best Success

When it comes to goal setting and meeting your challenges on your journey, research shows that the best successes come from believing you can reach your goal. Although in turn, reaching some goals, seeing and feeling achievement raises that belief. This is called self-efficacy. Professionals recommend interspersing some easier goals, or breaking down a larger goal into smaller parts.

Research continually points out that social support increases success in reaching goals. In one study, with participants in a weight program who did it alone, 76% completed the program and 24% kept off the weight loss for six months. However, for those with social support, 95% completed the program and 66% were able to keep their weight loss for six months.

Such support can even occur online. Several recent studies have shown that weight loss support via social networking using Facebook, Instagram or any number of specific weight loss "apps" can be very effective in helping to set and meet weight loss goals.

6
BEST PRACTICES
– WHICH APPROACH IS RIGHT FOR YOU?

"Ugh, be gone!"

If only my extra flab could just melt away with the wave of a magic wand! But instead, I have to deal with a mind-boggling choice of diet plans. And all I see vanishing into thin air are my favorite foods. All the good stuff - *poof, gone* - replaced with things I've hated, ever since my mom made me eat them, sitting there on my plate. Can I ever find a diet that's really made for me?

Yes, you can, and it doesn't take magic, or tricks, or gimmicks - it just takes good science!

Even though the weight loss industry takes in $60 billion annually on experts, coaches, companies, solid meals, liquid meals, supplements and diets that feature and specialize in just about every single kind of food or food group, scientific evidence shows that as many as 90% of dieters gain back the weight they lost within 1-2 years. And it's almost always for the same reason. "Quick weight loss" solutions do little to encourage the kinds of lifestyle changes proven able to lead to permanent weight loss.

Research, which has followed that minority of dieters who have achieved long-term and successful weight loss, reveals that it's not actually any *specific* diet method, but a couple of specific diet traits that lead to success:

1. How well you individualize a diet plan into your lifestyle.

2. What behavior strategies you have in place to fall back on when your "willpower" or stick-to-itiveness starts to waiver.

There are many diets making the rounds at all times, and new ones are always popping up. Here's a run-down on some of the more frequently discussed diets and diet concepts with some research-backed pros and cons.

But First, A Note About Mindfulness

Mindfulness is a complementary health approach being practiced as part of various weight loss programs. Recent evidence has shown that the mind/body approach of mindfulness is safe and helpful for weight loss. Much of the research and evidence with mindfulness techniques show positive results from using yoga exercise programs and eating practices. Not all of the diets listed incorporate mindfulness in their approach, but those that do tend to be more successful for long-term weight loss.

Hot Topic Diet Books and Plans

The Mediterranean Diet Book focuses on wholesome, unprocessed foods. There is a first phase of 10-days where you eliminate sugar and refined foods and focus on vegetables, lean protein, good fats, and whole grains. In the next stage you have a wide variety of foods and a tiny piece of dark chocolate 1-3 times a week and one glass of wine a day. In the third stage you learn to maintain weight loss.

There's no calorie counting, but portion sizes are used. The book also focuses on mindfulness in eating, to both enjoy and savor one's food. This results in helping participants manage portion control and choose healthier foods. Spokespeople for the Obesity Program at the University of Carolina state that eating this diet has proven in recent studies to improve health and weight loss. Other experts in weight loss agree that when people lower their sugar intake they usually don't want it or crave it as much.

The difficult part of this diet plan that could lead to disappointment and failure is cutting out potentially favorite foods, especially during the first week.

The Eating Every 3 Hours Diet was developed by registered medical professionals and is designed to keep metabolism going, burning fat while saving lean muscle, and stabilizing blood sugar. A daily plan for breakfast, snack, lunch, snack, dinner and treat is established. It limits calories to around 1,400 per day, does not limit all choices, but requires vegetables, healthy carbs, protein and good fat at each meal. This diet includes portion controls and suggestions for journal keeping and a support system for emotional eating difficulties. While there are no large studies that support these claims about metabolism raising that burns fat and not muscle, the American Dietetic Association offers that this plan helps people manage cravings and binges, since it allows any foods, in portion-controlled amounts, and provides advice on emotional eating. This diet also allows for flexibility - the three-hour time rule can be varied a bit, as long as reliance is on wholesome foods and portion control is adhered to.

The Inflammation Diet was created by health professionals. The diet is designed to reduce internal inflammation, which, as much recent evidence has shown, does help to reduce the risk of many diseases. The diet also claims to help people lose weight. There are calorie focused plans that provide dieters with options within a daily diet composed of about 50% carbs, 20% protein, and 30% fat. You are advised to eat inflammation-fighting foods from a list of over 1,500 items that have inflammation ratings for each. For example, vegetables are high while poultry is low. There is some research that shows a correlation between extra body fat and inflammation. There is also research showing that what you eat results in either anti-inflammatory or causal inflammatory substances to be active in the body. This diet is deemed to be healthy with good food choices and proportions by health experts; however, the results for losing weight quickly or in keeping it off in the long term have not proven to be great.

The Intermittent Fasting Diet is a plan that calls for you to eat what you want for five days, then over the next two days, you fast. There are many who have used it and claim they have steadily lost weight with an average loss of one pound a week. There is a lot of favorable talk about this diet because of quick weight loss. Since there is restraint for only two days a week, during the five other days participants find they do not have to be so concerned with dieting. They find the two day fast can fit into schedules.

On the other hand, it's not easy to go two consecutive days with not eating, and should be done only with health provider consultation for your own safety and body requirements. Professionals and research do indicate that just about any diet that restricts calories will result in initial weight loss, but the long-term challenge is maintaining those same diet restrictions in order to keep off the weight.

The South Beach Diet has been reported by many to help drop pounds relatively quickly, but little evidence as yet indicates this diet is one in which weight can be kept off for the long term.

There are diet programs and diet programs that are fads and quick fix diets. The diet industry often exploits, for their own monetary gain, dieter's feelings of shame and anticipation of desired, speedy satisfaction.

The Flat Belly Diet has not provided great evidence for either short or long term weight loss and it is believed its claims are exaggerated.

Professionals caution against plans that provide temporary dietary discipline. Once individuals move off packaged meals and back to regular eating and cooking, weight is likely to come back. For this reason, experts in nutrition deemed the following plans unhelpful for either short or long term weight loss: Flat Belly, Medifast, Nutrisystem, and Zone. Diets determined by experts as effective include: The Mayo Plan, TLC, Weight Watchers, DASH, and LEARN.

Fad Diets

Fad diets are often all about restricting caloric intake to far below what people usually eat daily. Nutritionists agree that most of these diets are not nutritionally balanced because, by excluding various food groups, they lack important nutrients the body needs and normally acquires from the wide range of food groups. Many times fad diets promote themselves with certain statements people need to be wary of, such as claiming 100% success or boasting possible weight loss of more than two pounds a week. Also, beware of diets that provide only personal testimonials without the back up of valid research.

Supplements

There are various supplements, often enzymes or vitamins, and various herbal products that are promoted as weight loss supplements. It's always advisable to check with a health care provider about the safety and/or actual effects of any of these on your unique body system.

Supplements, like fad diets, are often promoted with unrealistic, exaggerated descriptions. Be wary of claims that products are totally safe and quick and effective, as well as personal testimonials with no objective studies based on evidence. Be skeptical of endorsements by celebrities who have no background in fitness or nutrition. Always remember anything that sounds too good to be true, probably isn't true!

The following university-based studies with large samples and clinical trials indicate some weight loss strategies that have been proven to work.

1. Counting the Bites You Eat

In this study, the group that counted bites using a pitch counter lost more weight and felt satisfied more quickly than the group that ate as they normally would. This study supports other positive evidence using mindfulness methods of focus and attentiveness to the body's natural satiety (feeling of fullness) cues - which may be overshadowed in other circumstances by emotions and stress.

2. Eating a Good Breakfast

In this study, two groups ate the same amount of daily-restricted calories. The group that ate a 600 calorie breakfast that was protein rich and did include a small cookie, cake or doughnut lost more weight than those eating a meager 300 calorie breakfast of relatively little protein. The study determined that the larger substantial breakfasts helped participants stick to their daily calorie regimen and helped them be less tempted to stray or to eat junk food.

3. Exercising for 1/2 Hour

This study showed that individuals who did high impact exercise for 1/2 hour lost more weight than those doing the same high impact exercise for one hour. The researchers believe this is because those exercising for the longer period often compensated by straying from their diet plans and eating junk foods. Additionally, the longer period of exercise may have taken a toll on the dieter's storehouse of willpower.

4. Eating Your Vegetables

This study compared the low-carb Atkins diet, the healthful and legume-based Mediterranean diet, and a low-fat, high-carb diet plan. The participants on the low-carb lost the most weight and had the best success in maintaining the weight loss over two years. The amount of vegetables they ate was the most important factor in their weight loss. Researchers in this study explained that vegetables, which contain long-proven, important nutrients and fiber for every body, also seem to make a more of a positive difference in a diet, calorie for calorie, than other food groups.

5. The Importance of "Shut-Eye"

In this study, one group slept for up to nine hours a night over a period of several days while the other group was restricted to just four hours of sleep a night. You can probably already guess from your own experience that those with less sleep were more likely to stray from any weight loss program and eat junk food. The researchers explained with two reasons:

> 1. Sleep deprivation causes the body to desire a quick burst of energy and thus exhibit a preference for sugary foods and high fat foods, which are also usually sugary as well.
>
> 2. When not getting the proper amount of sleep needed by a normal brain for optimal function, the brain's abilities to avoid tempting and unhealthy behaviors is hampered.

6. The Long Haul Stick-to-itiveness

This study focused on what types of weight loss plans lead to successful results over two years or more. The study determined that the best plan is an individualized person's own choice of plan with foods that he or she enjoys which meet personal preferences and cultural norms, allergy requirements and overall lifestyle. Dieters with long-term successes are also bolstered by support from friends, nutritionists and psychologists who help with formulating methods for combating temptations and negative thoughts so that dieters persevere.

7. Support and Buddies

A study published in the *Journal of Consulting and Clinical Psychology* found better weight loss success when people exercise with a buddy who also is simultaneously involved in losing weight. The researchers explained that friends help to keep you accountable and honest. Friends give you support without barriers and provide motivation by offering encouragement.

Essentially, weight loss diets and plans must be suitable to you and your unique needs, your preferences, your lifestyle, your goals, and your behaviors.

Think about any previous diet plans you've tried and list what you already know about yourself and the successes or failures of those diet plans.

1. Did the plan work for you? Why or why not?

2. How did you feel physically and emotionally while on this diet?

3. Did you do it alone or with others for support? What did you like or not like about your level of independence and/or camaraderie?

4. Did costs for the plan fit in your budget?

5. Did you then or do you now have any health conditions, allergies, religious or cultural requirements, food preferences?

6. Do you like flexibility or very structured plans?

7. Do you like a variety of foods, or are limitations OK for you?

Whatever plans you are considering, make sure to choose one that will work best for you, one that is professionally recommended for a healthy lifestyle and long term results.

Make sure to choose a plan that includes:

1. Variety from your major food groups, including nutrient-dense vegetables, fruits, whole grains, lean protein, low fat dairy, nuts and seeds along with occasional sweet indulgences.

2. A good balance of nutrients and calories.

3. An enjoyable physical activity program to coincide with your diet plan.

The truth about fitness and long-term weight loss is that there is no magic secret, just simple common sense: *eat right and exercise*. The key is to find ways to accomplish this in ways that work for you, and only you, so that exercise becomes an enjoyable part of your everyday life, and your diet is focused on all the things you *get*, not what you *give up*.

This takes retraining your mind as much as your body, which you'll learn in the chapters ahead.

7
STRATEGIES FOR CONTROLLING YOUR EMOTIONAL TRIGGERS AND STRESS OVEREATING

"Oh fudge…and I mean it!"

That fudgy, creamy, ice cream or cake, the delectability of the cool whipped cream followed by that crunchy, salty bag of chips. *"Mmmm…it's calling my name, and here it goes into my mouth…there goes everything…oh my, oh dear…."*

Diet cheating, cravings, even lying to yourself about what it all means is often spurred on by certain pleasures. Emotional eating, cravings, and temptations that surround your life can imprison you with uncontrollable urges and actions.

What Triggers Emotional Eating?

A first wise step to understanding and controlling emotional overeating is to know what lurks behind your triggers. Call them out into the open, divide and conquer! There are ways to manage these triggers with various techniques. But first, let's look at some temptations that trigger binging and emotional eating as described by psychologists.

Social Eating

It's easy to want to eat along with others who are eating in order to join in, or to fit in. Often people who struggle with weight also struggle in social situations and crave the need to fit in, just as much as they crave sugar! Social situations can be a double whammy of temptations and easily trigger the desire to overeat within the setting, and/or to stray from set goals.

Emotions and Eating

We feel and hear other people verbally express these emotions all the time, "I'm bored." "I'm stressed out." "I'm tense." "I'm angry." "I'm so exhausted." "I'm anxious." "I'm lonely." Many try to either replace or cover up these emotions with food, and that can lead to overeating. These emotions can sap your strength and mental energy, getting in the between you and your goals.

Sometimes, even strong positive emotions inspire emotional eating as a reward or satisfaction. For example, you receive a fabulous job offer, or your fiancée accepts your proposal, and all too often a celebration occurs with something like a super-sized burger and a large shake. And that can just spiral into the fast food/ fat food addictions.

Emotional hunger usually comes on suddenly and you find yourself deeply craving certain foods, whether or not you're hungry, and whether or not it's a convenient or proper time or location for a meal.

Self Esteem Issues

People frequently determine that they've failed themselves. They become disappointed in their actions, reactions, or lack thereof. They feel as though they've dashed their own hopes, caused their own plans to not work out, and goals to remain unreached. The emotional response that follows is to scold and berate themselves, which is accompanied by feelings of unworthiness. Faltering self esteem, forgetting self worth in the face of normal human failures, causes many people to overeat for solace. Succumbing to temptations to soothe feelings of inadequacy, rather than simply forgiving themselves and moving on, is a common by-product of low self-esteem.

Spur-of-the-Moment Eating

Advertising bombards us. Restaurants and grab-and-go food stands are everywhere, not to mention our own pantries and refrigerator contents. Food is visible and promoted all around us. The opportunity to buy any type of food is omnipresent. Choosing to grab something you just happen to see as it strikes your fancy can push you off the path of your goals.

Rituals and Eating

It's the American way - hot dogs and beer at ball games, cotton candy and steak and pepper grinders and fried dumplings at county fairs, buttered popcorn and extra large candy and soda at movies, and absolutely anything in front of the TV. These rituals carry with them an allure, the notion that eating is the thing to do on certain occasions unrelated to meals. Associating these situations with food enjoyment can easily trigger temptations and cravings.

Physical Responses and Overeating

Everyone has over-committed schedules and many make the mistake of skipping healthy, nourishing meals in order to rush on to the next obligation. Scientific studies show that skipping meals can lower blood sugar, cause energy levels to plummet and easily stimulate the physical need for quick sustenance. All too often, this leads to grabbing something you crave and/or overeating out of an emotional response, rather than feeding yourself with logical reasoning, seeking to compensate for that hunger feeling of headache, dizziness, fatigue, etc.

Stress Eating

Research by the American Psychological Association revealed that about 1/4 of Americans will rate their stress level as very high - 80 or more on a 100 point scale.

This research explains what takes place in the body as a reaction to initial and continued stress. When you first experience stress, the brain responds with certain actions. A hormone is released in the brain, which tends to suppress appetite. Messages are sent to the adrenal glands that release another hormone, epinephrine, also known as adrenaline. Adrenaline works to trigger the body's flight or fight response to stress, preparing to act and run rather than sit and eat. When stress continues or increases, the adrenal glands go into further action and release the hormone cortisol, which causes an increase in appetite and could also increase one's motivation to eat. If the stress persists, the cortisol can stay elevated, thus continuing the appetite and motivations. Finally, when the stress ends, cortisol will decrease.

Other recent studies show a correlation between emotional or physical stress and increased food intake of fats and sugars. In one study with stressed mice, high carb foods were taken away from them resulting in an increase in their stress. In humans as well, fats and sugary foods - the "comfort foods" - actually do comfort on a chemical level. There is evidence that individuals with high levels of cortisol are more prone to snack in respond to stress.

Countering Stress

Anyone who's ever got caught up in the viscous cycle of binge eating for the quickly disappointing comfort it may provide knows deep down inside that there has to be a better way. What follows is a run-down of alternative stress-busting techniques for you to consider which ones might work into your individualized diet plan and overall balanced lifestyle.

Removal/Avoidance

Get rid of trigger foods - especially sugary and fatty foods - from your kitchen.

Healthy Self-Soothing

Psychologists often recommend reaching out to supportive friends, maintaining a regular exercise program, carrying out daily spiritual practices such as prayers and gratitude statements, watching motivational videos, pursuing hobbies such as bird watching, crafting, music, biking and other sports, gardening, yoga and tai chi. Filling one's life up with activities that pump you up leaves little room to fill your body with those trigger foods that bring you down.

The following three methods and strategies are most often recommended by health professionals for working through stress, and emotions:

Cognitive-Behavioral Therapy

This works to help people find and deal with negative thoughts and emotions.

Problem Solving

Finding alternative solutions to the stressor in your life, other that eating, to make you feel better.

Mindfulness and Meditation

This practice helps individuals fully pay attention to food and eating with complete sensory awareness. Being mindful can help you be aware of and prevent impulses. Mindfulness includes the strategy of allowing thoughts and emotions to come and go without judging them and instead focusing on awareness of the moment.

Binge Eating

Emotions don't just happen out of the blue, but develop from life-long experiences. Compulsive behavior can arise from early traumatic experiences, either conscious or repressed, as well as the less traumatic parts of one's upbringing and early family experiences. According to Harmony Grove, an eating disorders treatment establishment, binging on food is often a learned response stemming from certain emotions people initially experience while growing up. For example, internalizing a belief that one is shameful can cause a person to unconsciously seek out ways to express that shame in order to reenact the old familiar feeling. This is a complicated psychological process that brings repressed and/or old familiar feelings into the present via a binge on food and thus forces the binger to try to dealt with it in the present. If past personal issues have not been addressed, binge eating can also act as a self-medication to avoid re-experiencing any pain from the trauma. Thus a vicious cycle continues.

Harmony Grove also describes a deeper emotion that hides behind the boredom, which many people blame for their tendencies to binge - that being a lack of self-motivation, purpose, or passion in life. Therefore, the temporary joy and passion of eating food serves as a substitute or distraction from the bigger thing missing in life. Eating provides instantaneous gratification on several levels. If a person feels an overall lack of hope or doubts that there's anything positive to look forward to, reaching for food to fill the void becomes second nature.

Conversely, when people dwell in the static expectation that something important or valuable in the near future is bound to happen soon, often that something becomes an oppressively huge snack or meal. Thus, a person's empowerment to pursue more authentic fulfillment gets put on hold.

Mindless eating often results in eating a huge amount without realizing it - the whole bag of cookies, the whole bowl of popcorn, the whole anything that is in front of you at the moment. When a person finds oneself eating without being conscious of the choice to eat, or the texture and taste of each bite, and how the food is affecting his or her satiety, a binge could be on the brink of occurring.

Riding Out an Urge to Binge

Counselors recommend if one of your regular self-soothing activities is not available to you when you notice one of your emotional triggers that lead to overeating or binging, organize some healthy alternatives that will stall the urge for even a short time. Suggestions include to buy some time with an activity that is readily available, gives you pleasure, and/or make you feel a sense of accomplishment. Consider brushing your teeth, painting your nails, watering plants, organizing drawers or closets, doing puzzles or crosswords, changing your environment or atmosphere, having a quick stash of low calories vegetables or fruit. Activities will be discussed more in the pages that follow.

Changing Habits

You have the power to transform your habits into ones that enrich your life. Part of the process is understanding the how and why of stress and emotional overeating habits.

Trigger Diary

Keeping a daily food diary that is truthful and doesn't leave gaps helps to identify your triggers, according to psychology professionals. Record what and when you eat, what stresses, emotions or thoughts are part of each eating experience. You should be able to see what your own patterns are pretty quickly.

Planning to Do A Pleasurable Substitute Activity

One method that psychology counselors often recommend to people beginning to face their triggers is to list alternatives to those triggers and have them already in place, available for whenever the trigger situation should arise. The list is endless and depends totally on your own interests and availabilities.

The following alternative substitute activities are often used: reading, walking, jogging, taking a bath or shower, deep breathing exercises, playing cards or video games, communicating with a friend, gardening, or doing housework.

So then, you recognize your habits and you want to change them, but research also shows stress and anxiety can limit the control you have over your behavior and choices. Much behavior is driven by your biochemistry and your conscious attention to things around you.

The emotional brain is often stronger and takes precedence over the more rational, thinking brain. What this means is, despite your best intentions, you cannot positively change your habits until you find positive ways to deal with your stress!

A new survey by psychology experts suggest that habits undermine the strengths needed to instruct the brain on making lifestyle changes, especially if it is something you are not committed to with positive intentions.

For example, think back if, after you eat a cookie or small piece of cake or pie, you feel guilt emotions, and then eat the whole box of cookies or the whole cake, rationalizing that you already failed the goal or the diet plan? If you were only operating on rationality, you could evaluate the situation like this: just one cookie is only minimally going to affect my calorie and sugar plan for the day, but many more will not do. With just one, I can get right back on track.

This study reported that about 43% of those who want to manage their weight found emotional eating in this manner a roadblock.

Once you take careful note of your triggers you can begin to develop alternatives for yourself and make new healthy habits.

For example, if there is a front desk where you work, and on it sits a bowl of hard-to-resist candy, can you take a different route on your office treks for necessities? If you crave sweets in the morning, try a variety of sweet, natural fruit or dried fruit. Keep healthy alternatives within reach.

Many people who are trying to stick to a diet encounter hurdles like attending a birthday party. They blame that delicious looking hunk of frosted chocolate cake in front of them for cheating on their diet. But it is possible to just say no. Think of running on a track and leaping the hurdle. It is not easy at first, but it does come with consistent practice.

It's important to figure out your stressors and then take steps to deal with each one. For some it's a certain person who could be avoided on the job. If the job itself is too stressful, then the priority becomes switching jobs for the sake of your healthy life.

But, before you turn in your two-week resignation, remember those professionally recommended practices mentioned before, such as cognitive-behavior therapy, problem solving, and mindfulness.

Mindfulness Does Make a Difference

A recent study in the *British Journal of Health Psychology* addressed the effectiveness in using mindfulness in resisting sweets - namely chocolate. Mindfulness involves a purposely focused awareness of the present moment. In this study, participants were in three groups:

A cognitive diffusion group in which they were tested on changing the relationship with their thoughts by purposeful instructions to look at themselves as different and separate from their thoughts. Using a mindfulness strategy called the mind bus, each participant viewed him or her self as a bus driver, while the passengers were their thoughts. This group used the mind bus tool for five days, any time they had a chocolate temptation or craving

In the acceptance group, the participants had to effectively deal with their cravings by using urge surfing. They were to accept their feelings without effort to control them. They were to recognize and acknowledge feelings and ride them out on a surfboard.

In the control group, participants used relaxation strategy with a physical method of contracting then relaxing various body muscles.

All participants kept chocolate diaries to account for the amount of chocolates they ate from a bag they were given, as well as any additional chocolate.

The results after five days: The mindfulness group ate notably less chocolate from the bag and somewhat less additional chocolate than the other groups.

Researchers offered various explanations for the results, but felt the success of the mindfulness methods primarily resulted from giving the participants a tool to overcome the habitual automatic chocolate eating that stemmed from emotional reactions to stress.

Psychology experts suggest using a mindfulness strategy at home whenever thoughts of the candy or cookie that are the urge come up. Be the bus driver of your urges, the passengers, and drive yourself to a healthy place on your path to your goal.

You can find out much more about mindfulness and weight loss in my companion book, co-authored with Cynthia Lechan-Goodman, *Mind Your Own Fitness*.

8
LIFESTYLE CHANGES IN FOOD AND NUTRITION

A large chocolate chip cookie for brunch! Preposterous?

No, because many have and do opt for a planned "cheat" day, or five days of a large chocolate chip cookie for brunch as a means of cutting calories and food intake in order to lose weight. Trouble is, they find soon enough, around a couple of hours after a cookie (or other treat) meal, that they feel hunger, lethargy, malaise set in and often wind up eating again or overeating as compensation.

All the recent studies and evidence show that it is exactly what you choose to eat, and how you eat that makes all the difference in weight loss and maintenance, and to be sure, one large cookie a day will have the opposite effect of weight loss.

Countless recent studies of food, eating, and weight discuss how nutritional components of foods effect your total body, and how much of these nutritional components are needed in a body's daily eating routines and eating plans. Countless studies also illuminate exactly what the nutritional components of an individual food are and the potential effects to your body when you eat that particular food item. So, it's great information for you to learn as much as you can about foods, and make plans for your daily eating lifestyle as you see fit, and you'll also see a body that is more fit.

Of course, there is so much food news, that it is often hard to pick and choose. You can hear bad news and confusing news about foods, such as the reports that carbs are fattening, or just eat carbs, warnings that fats are unhealthy, and be sure to eat healthy fats, caution about too much protein can harm your heart, or eat mostly protein, or eat only plant protein, be sure to add supplements, and watch out because supplements can have serious side affects.

Whew! Luckily, here are ways to clue you in, and help you be on top of lifestyle choices for eating - at home, out, on the run, on the job, and while snacking.

The Up-To-Date Food Plate

The government, with First Lady Michelle Obama in the lead, has offered a new image and way to plan your daily food to meet nutritional requirements. Gone is the pyramid, replaced by a serviceable dinner plate. The plate is nicely divided into four sections of different sizes, according to how much of each food group is recommended: the largest is for vegetables, a slightly smaller section for fruits, but the vegetables and fruits together make up 1/2 the plate. The second largest spot is for grains, and the smallest section is proteins which include meat, tofu, beans. There is a nice side dish also showing a smaller serving of dairy, which includes milks, cheeses, and yogurt.

When making up your fruit and veggie sections, choose a rainbow. Choose vibrant colors, which, according to recent plant science, indicate the foods are packed with good nutrients.

The guidelines have advisories on limiting sugar especially sugary drinks. Experts find that phasing out sugar will improve health, stabilize moods and energy levels, and actually give you the pleasures of tasting natural whole foods, and healthier foods.

There are naturally and healthier ways to please your sweet tooth than refined sugars and processed sweeteners such as high fructose corn syrup. Choosing natural sweeteners such as stevia, honey, maple syrup, agave, and fresh fruit in their wonderfully ripe stages will make a difference.

Many vegetables also are naturally sweet such as yams, carrots, and beets. Even natural grains and complex carbs can release a natural sweetness. Eating natural fruits and vegetables and complex carbs will also help to satisfy sugar cravings and curb excess sweet eating. And once you get your body to "remember" what natural sweetness tastes like, you will find that you will no longer even enjoy the taste of your former sweet cravings. Many, who have kicked the cookie, cake, and candy habit, describe these treats as tasting "sickeningly sweet" if they ever indulge. How right they are!

Nutritionists describe phasing out sugar as an act of self-care and self-love instead of punishment or deprivation. This is not easy, though. Studies at Princeton have shown how breaking a sugar habit is a formidable challenge, as there is evidence to suggest that sugar can be physically addicting much like cigarettes or alcohol. Another recent study indicated that there are similarities between sugar as an addiction and other bodily addiction responses. Researchers believe it involves dopamine, a hormone linked to pleasure and motivation. Overweight people, it is believed, have fewer receptors for dopamine and therefore may need more of sweet food to interpret the pleasure from it. Like other addictions, sugar consumption leads to increased use, withdrawal, cravings and relapse. Breaking a sugar habit is a challenge, not only because of its addictive qualities, but because it is everywhere - not just in desserts, but in breads, condiments, and soups.

When cutting down on sugar, you need to be aware of the hidden sugars in products. Sugar is in many things you may not realize, and even if you read the labels, it is not always listed as "sugar." Look for anything ending in "ose" or "tol" as these could be sources of hidden sugars.

Proteins, Carbohydrates and Fats

Medical professionals always recommend making sure your diet has a variety of foods. This is the best way for your body to receive the many essential nutrients you need to thrive. The body's everyday processes run on various nutrients: carbohydrates, proteins, fats, fiber, vitamins and minerals.

Carbohydrates include starches and sugars that break down to glucose, which is what body cells need for energy and power. Carbs are the body's main fuel. Some extra carbs are also stored in the liver for use at a future time when it is needed, but the liver only has a certain limit to how much it can store, and after the limit, the body turns extra carbs to fat. Almost all foods contain carbohydrates except for meat, poultry, eggs and some seafood.

Carbohydrates are classed into complex, or healthy carbs, and simple sugar carbs. Healthy carbs such as multi-grains, lentils, legumes, brown rice, vegetables and fruits, raise blood sugar slowly and last longer as opposed to simple or fast acting carbs such as cookies, cake, candy, soda, or juice, which raise blood sugar quickly and do not last very long. There are 4 calories to 1 gram of carbohydrates.

Fiber is a carbohydrate but it does not break down into glucose. It functions in the body's digestive tract to help manage and keep waste flowing and pushed out, and allows nutrients to be absorbed into your body through intestinal walls.

Fats are a major part of cells and blood vessels, and have a major role in the body's absorption of vitamins. They also contribute to body energy. If the body runs out of glucose, fats are also used for energy. Fats have 9 calories per gram. Fats do not have an effect on blood sugar, but if eaten together with carbohydrates they can slow blood sugar down, slow digestion, and keep blood sugar levels higher for longer lengths.

Fats are classed into mono-unsaturated and poly-unsaturated, which include olive, canola, nut and avocado oils. These are considered healthy because they lower LDL in the blood. Saturated fats such as meat and dairy product fats, palm oils and hydrogenated oils can damage arteries and the heart. Trans fats found in processed and fried fast foods also contribute to body damage. New information is coming to light about coconut oils being better for one's health than once thought, in regard to its effect on cholesterol levels.

Proteins are necessary for the very structure of all cells, for growth, maintenance and energy. They are used for energy if carbohydrates and fats are not available, and aids in lean muscle development. Proteins take a longer time to affect blood sugar levels, three to four hours, and the rise in blood sugar is relatively low.

Nutrients are substances in all foods that work in the body to perform all daily functions. Many of the healthy carbs, certain proteins, and fats are also termed super foods as they are considered loaded with nutrients It is the nutrient value of foods that makes for a lifestyle of health, vigor, well-being and abilities to sustain a weight loss plan and weight control/ maintenance.

Generally, your body knows what is good for it, and the nutrients that are needed for peak performance. But, your *mind* has a way of tricking you and your body into making bad food choices. But, you can retrain your brain just like rebooting your computer, by adding some new software!

Your Diet Reboot: What to Keep and What to Toss

If you analyze the food news out there, you might notice that it is fruits and vegetables that are always on the "nice" list. Rarely, if ever, will you see any diet plan that says, "You need to cut down on your fruits and veggies." There are libraries full of evidence that increasing your consumption of fresh fruits and vegetables, particularly those classified, as "super foods" are the surest way to reach your weight loss goals, and improve your overall, long-term health.

Protein and carbs have been studied and the importance has been revealed of keeping them both in your diet, in good balance. Eating proteins in excess often leads to cravings of excessive sweets. Not enough protein and there can also be sugar cravings. Vegetarian lifestyle eating plans have been touted by research because this type of diet relies on, in addition to veggies, whole grains and beans, which can offer a healthy balance of protein and carbs if developed properly.

The glycemic index (or GI) is a tool that is often valuable for people to understand some of the nutritional effects of foods, namely the effects of carbohydrates on the body. This tool ranks carb-containing foods based on how they raise blood glucose: foods measuring 70-99 are classified as high and include baked potatoes, watermelon, and graham crackers. Medium GI foods between 56-69 include whole-wheat items, brown rice, sugar, soda, and cheese pizza. Low GI range of 55 or less includes most fruits and vegetables, pasta, milk, pumpernickel bread, and legumes.

Research studies indicated that participants following a high protein, low glycemic index diet lost an average of .8 pounds after 26 weeks, while other groups gained an average of .7-3.7 pounds. Participants who used a low protein diet gained an average of two pounds more than the high protein diet, and participants who ate high glycemic foods gained two pounds more than those eating low glycemic foods. The researches felt one reason was the feeling of satisfaction that accompanies a high protein, low glycemic index diet is what enabled people to stick with it.

An intense, well-lived, healthy and fit life, which leads to good weight practices, is about getting the most out of each meal - well-balanced with the right amount of proteins, fats, carbs, nutrients, and vitamins. A good nutrient value per calorie ensures that you rebuild and repair your body systems optimally.

Portions and Portion Control

Portions, the servings people eat from packaged foods, restaurants, and even at home, have gotten out of control, and grown IMMENSELY over the past years.

America's "super-size" obsession is a main reason, research has proven, that contributes to weight gain and difficulties in losing and maintaining weight. For example, a soda serving used to be 6 ounces and 85 calories. Nowadays, it is usually 20 ounces and 300 calories. A standard bagel was 3 inches in diameter and contained about 140 calories, but now bagels are five to 6 inches and 350 calories.

A serving of pasta was 2 cups at 280 calories, and is now 4 cups at over 560 calories. A small order of fries was 230 calories, and now a large order is 500 calories with double the fat. Dinner plates were once 10 inches and are now 12 ½ inches.

A fast food burger in 1955 was, amazingly, just 1.6 ounces of meat compared to today's 8 ounces of 590 calories or so.

No WONDER we're fat!

General portion recommendations from the Baylor College of Medicine advise these measurements to keep in mind:

1 cup of food is the size of a baseball, or smaller fist, and foods measured by the cup include fresh greens, yogurt, fruit, and a baked potato.

One-half a cup of food is about a rounded handful and is a suggested normal portion of cut fruit, cooked vegetables, rice or pasta.

1 ounce of food such as snack foods like pretzels is also a rounded handful.

1/4 cup of almonds is about the size of a golf ball.

1/4 cup of food is the size of 1 large egg and this is often a measure of dried fruit such as raisins.

3 ounces of food is a suggested measure of items such as poultry, meat, or fish, and is about the size of a checkbook.

1 1/2 ounces of food such as the suggested serving size for cheeses is about the size of six dice.

1 ounce of food, or the size of one die is a good measure for fats such as butter and spreads.

1 tablespoon, which is the size of your thumb top, is suggested for oils, and mayo.

Resizing Tips

- Because grocery shopping today makes you buy large bags and portions, divide the contents of your packages into smaller, meal-sized portions before storing them in the pantry.

- Ask for half of your meal to be put in a "doggie bag" before it is served to you in a restaurant. This prevents overeating.
- When eating at home, use smaller plates. Your portions will have the visual effect of a full plate.

Food Myths and Pitfalls

Don't get suckered in by food myths. Check labels to determine if a food advertised as low fat, fat free, or low calorie is really worthwhile. Low fat or fat free products may not be low in calories. A bag of marshmallows proudly emblazons its label with "Fat-Free Food," but you don't see them on too many healthy diet plans! Often, these foods contain added, undesirable ingredients to make up for the flavor and texture of fats and add more calories.

The notion that skipping breakfast will subtract calories from your day is an erroneous belief. Research shows skipping breakfast leads to eating more than usual later in the day. Those people who don't eat breakfast have been studied, and are shown to be more overweight than those who eat a healthy breakfast. Short on time? Pack your breakfast the night before.

Good and Bad Foods

A recent study by the Harvard School of Public Health indicates that in the United States, our "diet is even worse" (than lack of physical activity), as a root cause of obesity and poor health. This corroborated a published study in *The New England Journal of Medicine* on the existence of good and bad foods and the advice to eat good foods more, and bad foods less. Researchers found that the kinds of foods people ate had a large effect on their overall lifestyle, health, and weight. The study showed that small changes in eating and other habits could result in large body weight changes over the years. The participants studied normally gained about a pound a year and 20 pounds in 20 years. Some gained 4 pounds a year.

Foods that produced the most weight gain were:

- French fries were linked to an average gain of 3.4 lbs. in every 4 years
- Potato chips were linked to a weight gain of 1.7 lbs.
- Sugary drinks accounted for 1 lb.
- Red meat and processed meat added .93 to .95 lbs.

Those foods that led to weight loss or maintenance were fruits, vegetables, and whole grains. Those who lost weight ate three or more servings of vegetables every day.

Dairy products did not show significant effects of either gain or loss on weight, except for two particular fats - eating yogurt and nut butters such as peanut butter. Participants who ate more yogurt and nuts such as peanut butter lost the most weight every four years.

Researchers believe the yogurt's results are due to healthy bacteria that may raise certain hormones in the intestines that increase satisfaction and decrease hunger.

Super Foods are Super

Certain foods and food groups have been termed "super foods" because they contain larger than average amounts of nutrients, vitamins and minerals, antioxidants, as well as their amounts of nutrients compared to their caloric content, thus they are also referred to as nutrient dense foods.

Additionally, each super food has specific nutrients that are unique to them, and are unique to their particular work and effect in your body.

The more super foods you eat, the better equipped you will be to build a stronger body, boost your immune system, and add energy and well being to your daily life, which in turn will contribute to your general attitudes about dieting and maintaining your weight.

Research has been conducted on almost every food category and type, determining genetic structures and micro substance components that make up the food, and then, how these components actually affect the body in all its systems and functions.

The extensive positive results and indications of these super foods show that by making these foods a part of your normal eating plan, you can change your biochemistry to a more healthy course, fending off body changes that lead to diseases, aging, and weight gain.

Eating super foods in your daily diet is one way to ensure you have optimum energy. When your energy level is great, you can feel more inspired to keep your diet on tract.

There are many super foods and nutrient rich foods; many of them are ones you probably already use.

Here is a run-down of the super foods and what makes them so heroic:

Dark berries, such as blueberries, strawberries and boysenberries, salmon, sardines, leafy green vegetables, cruciferous vegetables, oranges and citrus fruits and pineapples.

Most of the super foods are also very high in fiber. Research has shown that a diet high in fiber helps with weight loss and weight management. Pritikin Longevity Center recommends 25 grams daily of fiber, but studies show that most American women eat only about 1/3 that amount. Whole grains, beans, fruits and vegetables are all good sources with many specific super foods in those groups rated high in fiber.

Chia seeds are often on the super food list, and they are a powerhouse of fiber. They are easy to use - just toss them into drinks or smoothies, and eat them along with most any food.

Almonds are usually on every super food listing, with their wonderful combination of protein, fiber, vitamins and minerals. In a study at Loma Linda University, dieters who ate almonds daily lost 62% more weight and 56% more fat than those who didn't.

Pine nuts boast excellent nutrients as well as being helpful in weight loss. Pine nuts contain pinolenic, a type of fat that produces hormones in germs called cholecystokinin and glucagons peptide which research has shown are involved in sending the brain signals that you are satiated. Eating pine nuts may result in a helpful appetite reduction. In one study, the participants ate 36% less when including 1 1/2 ounces of pine nuts in a daily diet plan.

And yes, you may have heard correctly – chocolate is a super food. BUT only the "real" dark chocolate containing at least 80% cacao, and only in moderation.

Purchasing Healthy Foods and Groceries

Losing weight is big business. You will continually see new and exciting "diet foods" on display or in the weekly circulars of your favorite food stores. Usually, they are nicely packaged for convenience and displayed for hard to resist value and often, if you try them, they don't taste bad. They may even taste rather good, and you may even lose a pound or so using them - at first that is.

But these products are not generally recommended for continual weight loss. If you review the nutritional content on their labels, you will see that most have artificial ingredients - chemicals, and processed additives that have little nutritional value for their calories. Diet foods often contain large amounts of sugar and salt, added to make up for the fats and sugars that are removed. Unfortunately, because of the taste value and the convenience value and the expected weight loss results, nutritional experts believe this can lead to a type of addiction - a continuance to use these products and foods, over healthier natural food choices.

Nearly everyone wants and needs convenience foods, and if you have freezer space, you can create your own "convenience food." Make extras of healthy meals you prepare at home, and freeze them in meal-sized portions for a quick lunch or dinner.

You can never go wrong buying the most natural products you can - organic, if possible. Whole grains, organic lean meats and poultry, fruit and vegetables, real yogurts such as Greek yogurts that are not heavily sugared, unprocessed cheeses, low fat milk, soy milk or almond milk.

You do not have to eliminate treats, but buy desserts and packaged foods in moderation.

Restaurant Savvy for Eating Healthy

A lot of people think that dieting for a healthier lifestyle means never going out to eat again! Not true. Many a "foodie" is at his or her optimal weight and in good shape, because they know how to eat out and really enjoy the experience!

It is a good plan to look over your menu choices and consider whether or not you really need a complete, four-course meal from appetizer to desert. Think ahead about your portions and put them all on your plate in your mind. If you pile a plate of soup, appetizer, salad and dressing, a couple of rolls and butter, a main course, two sides, a dessert, wine, a beverage and coffee, you can already see how high the pile is on the plate, and you can imagine the calories, fats, and sugars you will have eaten. That is not to say you can't enjoy something from each category, but diet experts recommend cutting your portion size in half, and boxing up half of what is served before you begin to eat.

For reduced calories and optimal health, choose grilled or broiled over fried and sauced. In selecting sauces, choose tomato rather than cheesy.

For alcohol, choose a single glass of red wine or light beer, which has health value. Mixed drinks, however, often have high amounts of extra sugar.

Natural fruit desserts are best, of course, or a low fat selection. But if that isn't an option, plan to share a dessert, and/or box it up before digging in. And of course, avoid the "all you can eat buffets," except on very rare, very special occasions!

Home Food Supplies

Planning a weekly nutritional and balanced menu for your meals at home is always recommended to avoid the urge to pounce on fast foods or quick food fixes to tide you over outside your home.

A good place to start is online at www.whfoods.com. The World's Healthiest Foods, a non-profit foundation, offers scientifically substantiated, easy to read information for convenient and enjoyable healthy eating.

Essential nutrients are nutrients that your body can't make on its own. How these nutrients are introduced into your body can influence how well your body can use them.

Nutrients do not work alone but along with other nutrients. Your body can benefit getting your nutrients from eating fresh whole foods because they give you the best and most of individual nutrients but also the variety necessary for their optimal function.

Eating Methods

Most of us eat quickly and may not even notice how quickly or how much we are eating, and many times, what is even on the plate! Here are some suggestions from health professionals to help you slow down.

After each bite, put your fork or spoon down for a minute rather than keeping up a nonstop motion. This way you bite, chew, taste, swallow and then pick up the utensil again. You experience each part of the process.

When you chew and swallow, make sure to swallow each bite, each mouthful before taking another bite, rather than loading your utensil and preparing to eat while still chewing and swallowing. Relax before beginning to eat with breathing exercises, prayer, meditation, something light to read, or by listening to music. Calm yourself and be fully present before you begin to eat.

Use courses for your meals, rather than placing all the food on the table at the same time. This allows for additional relaxation and breathing time.

Use a timer, if necessary. Take a little break once or twice during a meal by talking, sipping a beverage, or just sit listening with hands folded. Studies have indicated that listening to music during a meal helps to slow down eating.

When you are preparing food for a meal, resist tasting some until you are seated at the table to eat. There can be no accounting for how many of these tastes add up to a meal in itself!

Use chopsticks, which can slow movements from plate to mouth compared to the rate of fork to mouth.

Eat sitting down. Often people eat standing, in the car, on the run and are not even aware of this food as part of their daily intake and therefore are not accounting for it on their diet plans.

Make a meal a pleasurable event. When you eat, your brain will receive signals from your body, stomach and intestines to let you know you are full. However, it takes about 20 minutes for signals to travel from your lower body to your brain, so that eating too quickly can mean you eat extra food, mouthfuls of calories more than your body needs before your body is ready to give you the full signal. When you eat leisurely and relax, your brain will be able to register when you are full so that you can stop.

Enjoy your food with your senses. Your bodily sense of satisfaction is shown in research to be aided by taking the time, the awareness, the mindfulness of your food in order to experience it with your senses of smells, textures, appearance, as well as with taste sensations.

Tips for Eating Pleasure and Weight Loss

Mindfulness methods are great habits to develop because they help you understand and develop skills for listening to your body's cues about your state of hunger or fullness.

1. First, make sure you're not in autopilot eating mode.

2. Check out your hunger on a scale of 1-10 and ask yourself if you are physically hungry or not.

3. Notice if you have critical thoughts such as "I'm stupid, I'm an idiot to do that." Studies have shown that critical thoughts can trigger overeating. Mindfulness methods have been shown to help ease each critical thought before it influences your emotions and actions to eat. Harvard University researchers have studied results that suggest a slower, more thoughtful and aware mode of eating could help with many of the problems associated with overeating, including stress and making healthy food choices.

4. Try to avoid eating while multitasking so that any snack breaks or meal breaks you take are only about what is on your food plate and not which to-do lists may also be filling up your plate.

5. Developing mindful eating methods that give you pleasure, joy, and the excitement of an eating experience will help you meet your weight goals.

Paying Attention to Eating

Of course everyone relishes eating, and there is often great fun in the spontaneity involved in feeling like something, and eating it. Study after study has shown, though, that paying close attention to what you eat helps to keep track of serving sizes, health benefits and overall weight loss and maintenance goals.

Food journaling is one recommended procedure that requires dieters to make informed choices. Study researchers said when people write down what they eat, they have to think about it, so it can more often be seen as a treat. This helps in reaching weight loss goals.

Mindful Bites

Most of us have had the experience of eating something and not remembering those bites. You can be mindful by bringing all your senses to your eating experience. Breathe in the aromas of a meal being prepared, or the food sitting in front of you, or even a single bite before you put it in your mouth. What do the smells feel like going through your nose and enveloping you? Notice the colors, the appearance, and the textures of the food. Experience the nuances of colors on just one piece. What does the texture feel like on your tongue as you chew? Taste each bite as you chew slowly, letting all four of your tongue's taste bud areas have a chance to register the tastes - often there are more than one in each bite of food.

70-75% of what people perceive as taste is really from your sense of smell detected as odor molecules that travel between your nose and mouth to the brain. Your brain then gets the signals of the scent. A person normally discriminates between 4,000-10,000 odor molecules. Science discovered that odor is only detected in a liquid form so breathing takes either odor vapors or combines odor molecules with mucus moisture to transmit the information to your brain.

The Importance of Chewing

Each food is a mixture of different molecules of nutrients. The human body functions from a variety of types of nutrients, and complex combinations of nutrients. How each nutrient is digested will effect how your body uses them.

Chewing, also called mastication, is needed to break down large clumps of food molecules into smaller parts and combine those with your saliva and mouth enzymes.

Chewing is really the first stage of digestion, which sends the signal to your nervous system and brain to start the process.

The tastes of food trigger the stomach lining to produce acid. Saliva helps to improve the chewing process and begins the breakdown of carbs and fats. It takes about 1/2-2 hours for food to travel through the stomach and continue throughout the digestion process for an additional two to six hours, and then spending between 6-72 hours in the large intestine before elimination of waste.

Incomplete digestion means not all the nutrients in the food get absorbed by the body, which can result in extra food not absorbed causing bacterial overgrowth, gas and indigestion.

Digestion is a complex process because food is complex. Every food is made up of molecules that can be proteins, carbs, fats, vitamins, minerals or phytonutrients, and the molecules of each of these are different sizes, and need different processes in your digestion.

The work of the teeth as they grind up and chew is what begins the digestion process, and this does not happen the way it should if you are distracted while eating, and not attuned to appreciating and savoring your food. When you are relaxed and mindful of your eating, your body is in parasympathetic mode, which means it is totally attentive and ready to best digest your food.

Digestion and getting the nutrition and energy you need from food may be an unconscious process, but you consciously influence it by what you eat and how you eat it.

Just like when it comes to cars and computers, it's the same with your body. "Garbage in - garbage out." The choice is yours!

9
LIFESTYLE CHANGES: ACTIVITIES AND EXERCISE

"Move it, move it" was a ditty from a hit song a while back, and encouraged many to shake a tail feather, just one of the hundreds of perfect ways to include the activity of all-important exercise in your daily life. All health professionals, backed by extensive studies do show that physical activity and/or exercise is necessary if you are looking for weight control, weight loss, and/or maintenance of weight loss.

The Harvard School of Public Health recently published a study in *The New England Journal of Medicine* showing that physical activity, as expected, did show benefits for weight control. In fact, participants who exercised *less* gained weight, while those who exercised more did not, and those who increased their activity the most *gained almost two pounds less than all the others in four years.*

So, with any new musical number that has a good beat, get yourself up off the comfy couch, and get ready for more information to help lift your spirits - and booty - into the whys and hows of making room for physical movement in your daily life style.

Get With the Program

Programs for exercise and/or activities such as any sports classes or leagues - at home or at a facility - have plentiful statistics backing their helper status with successful weight loss/weight management and weight maintenance.

The support you can gain from being in a program with others who have similar goals is cited as one of the major reasons for a program's success in a healthy lifestyle. Many facilities and programs provide, either on-site, or online for weight loss eating plan along with the activities and exercises, a maintenance plan, and/or personal support from a group or buddy system, or even a dietician.

Motivation for Exercise

List all your goals you'd like to gain from exercise such as losing weight, reducing fat, building muscle, improvement in a sport, ability to join in sports and activities comfortably with family and friends.

Monitoring your own goals and progress will keep you aware both of your goals and your daily input and help to keep you on the right track.

Finding someone to exercise with, especially another person who is also looking to lose weight, helps with continuity and encouragement.

Health professionals all recommend that for best motivation, continuance, and maintenance, you need to shake it up while you are shaking it off, and vary your types of activities. Mix it up with more than one sport or class. Different activities also give you total body fitness potential, the opportunity to socialize with more people and potentially adding to your buddy support.

Research evidence supports the idea that people who exercise not only to lose weight, but who exercise doing an activity they truly enjoy, leads to better results in sticking to it. Remember exercise is not only for your body; it's for your mind too!

Research has shown that many of the positive results from regular exercise occur because exercise helps to reduce stress levels, and it has also been found that exercising outdoors reduces stress the most.

Make sure you don't lose the momentum, impetus and repetition of developing a good exercise habit by missing exercise sessions. If it happens, make up for it that week, or as soon as possible, or plan on a substitute activity you can easily fit in at home.

Give yourself ample rewards.

Yes, it's easy to stall, to just imagine a long winding road, an uphill battle, and all those defeatist slogans. Use a positive slogan and don't throw in the towel. Know that daily exercise will not deplete your energy, but give you an increased, improved and steadier flow of energy throughout your day. And if you combine your activity and exercise list with outdoor activities, you'll find new personal pleasures and appreciations for your environment.

Weight loss will come if you keep on keeping at it. The point is, you have to change your mindset towards exercise. Stop thinking about it as something "you need to do to lose weight," but just something that is a natural part of your everyday life. When you do that, the weight loss just happens.

Gyms

If you don't already have a gym or health club membership, try out those in your area. Research what they have available for activities and exercises that you might enjoy. Make sure they are held at a time and location that is convenient for you. Can you easily get there on time from work or from home? Check out these facilities during the times of the day that you're actually considering going there to workout to see how you feel about the crowds, the staffing, the traffic, etc.

Before you go, make a list of the activities you like or think you might like to try, and those you know you don't like so you have in mind a good picture of your real interests.

Many health clubs offer a free tour, class visit and/or trainer evaluation.

The Gym Embarrassment

Some people worry - a lot - about how they look to others (and themselves). But gyms are filled with both those who show off the products of long and continued work with chiseled and muscular bodies, and also awkward and out of shape beginners trying to lose weight, and improve their fitness. People new to exercise tend to be self-conscious around almost every one. It's a matter of just getting used to the routines and environment. Eventually you'll stop worrying over it because the truth is, every person is self-conscious to some degree and involved with themselves. They don't leave much room to be worrying about or judging you.

Stick-to-itiveness

Researchers and health professionals all agree the most optimal way to help yourself in a weight loss/ maintenance program with activity and exercise, is to not miss a workout that you have put into your daily/weekly plans. Keeping an exercise or activity diary, week by week, does have much researched evidence to back up its helpfulness in encouragement and successes. Of course, family and work and occasional illnesses do occur, which require changes in your exercise plans, but the pros advise to make up for it on another day, or make your next session longer to compensate. Prepare an emergency at-home make-up set of exercises as a substitute for those inevitable necessary missed workouts at the gym. The types of activities many people choose to do at home include working out to exercise videos. Consider designing one yourself with the music of your choice.

Choosing Activities

On any given day, there is a plentiful array of activities around your home and life in general that qualify as exercise - even if you can't join a gym, class or program, and if you don't need have space for exercise equipment.

Walking briskly, even for 10 minutes at a time, is helpful. Walk from home to parking lots, to bus stops, do gardening, join a walking group, walk to the shopping mall, walk the dog rather than watching him. Push that stroller; join in the kids with their soccer or bike rides. Even if you are watching a game, walk the sidelines. Clean house, wash the car, jump into the raked leaves, put on rain boots and be a kid and splash in the puddles, get your mojo on and dance. Replace coffee breaks with a 10-minute walk. Bat tennis balls against a wall. Go on nature hunts with the kids.

The important thing is to make activity part of your daily living...and make your days chock full of activities that you enjoy and that get you moving. Keep an extra set of clothes and shoes where you work or in the car to use on the spur of the moment.

Government Guidelines and Statistics

To maintain a healthy weight, government guideline recommendations are to exercise five times a week to the point where your heart rate is raised significantly.

Research indicates that the stresses of life today contribute to fattening people up. Researchers theorize that stressful events cause people to crave single carb snacks to calm stress hormones. Prehistorically, stress meant the body's energy would surge to enable the body to run from danger. But today, people's stresses are not run from, literally, but are experienced usually sitting down. So, using simple carbs to ameliorate stresses, aren't being used and the extra calories translate to extra lbs.

One study showed that stressed mice became even more stressed if their carbohydrate high foods were taken away - their stress hormones surged.

Recommendations are to exercise to the intensity level where you reach the point of sweating and breathing heavily.

A recent *American Journal of Health Promotion* study reveals that just a few minutes of any type of brisk physical activity each day can all add up and count as protection against obesity. Less than 5% of adults do the recommended levels of physical activity in a week. The National Health and Nutrition Exam survey recommendations for adults are 150 minutes of moderate to vigorous activity each weak. Vigorous exercise is determined as a level comparable to walking in a room at three miles per hour. To maintain weight, recommendations are that you need to do 30 minutes of moderate exercise each day, increasing to a level that raises your heart rate and causes you to break into a light sweat, five days a week. If your BMI is greater than 23, you might need to increase the intensity of the exercise.

In another recent study by the University of Utah, participants who performed higher intensity and short duration exertion showed benefits to their body mass index. Women who spent one more minute of high intensity exertion every day had a .07 decrease in their body mass, and for every extra minute every day of high intensity exertion, their odds for obesity decreased by 2-5%.

Is Exercise as Important as Diet?

Both are important, according to all studies and health professionals. But statistics show that exercise helps in both losing weight, and keeping those well-earned results ongoing and part of lifestyle. The National Weight Control Key study showed, that of people who lost at least 30 pounds and kept it off for at least one year, 90% exercised regularly, many by just brisk walking.

A new study by the University of Copenhagen published in the *American Journal of Physiology* showed that after 13 weeks, participants who had no change in diet or a sedentary lifestyle had no change in body fat. Participants who exercised and worked out for 60 minutes a day burning 600 calories in jogging, or cycling sweating, lost an average of five pounds. The participants who exercised moderately for 30 minutes a day burning 300 calories lost about 8 pounds. Researchers revealed that food diaries of those exercising one hour and burning 600 calories reported increasing their meals and snacks and calorie intake and were sedentary and felt fatigued outside of the exercise program. Those with moderate 1/2 hour exercise were inspired and energized and still active following and before exercise.

Researchers interpret their results as meaning that shorter sessions burn calories without people feeling the urge or need to replace those calories. The longer, more strenuous sessions were more draining and created more of a desire to fill up lost energy stores. One possibility, the study determined, is that strenuous exercise which puts on muscle actually contributed to the measure of weight loss by losing fat and gaining muscle on the shorter durations. In the long run, though, added muscle could raise metabolism and further the weight loss.

Metabolism - The Complex Consideration

So much has been learned and so much is still to be learned about what affects weight loss. A new study reveals that the American diet over the years has changed our brain, damaging the signaling pathways in the part of the brain that regulates metabolism - the hypothalamus. This study reported in the *British Journal of Nutrition* revealed that eating fattening foods has been shown to cause inflammation of cells going to the hypothalamus, overloading the neurons and causing neurological damage.

In another study from the University of Liverpool, a diet high in saturated fat and simple carbs set in motion a chain reaction of metabolic dysfunction involving appetite regulating hormones leptin and ghrelen. Leptin's job is to suppress appetite while ghrelin's job is to increase it.

Also, fatty high carb diets resulted in brain changes, alterations from too many calories from fat and simple sugars damaging nerves that conduct signals through the hypothalamus, affecting the leptin and ghrelin and the body's ability to regulate weight and metabolism. The signals don't get to the brain that might say you have enough fat stored already, so the person feels empty all the time, even when full.

The researchers believe some damage may be permanent but believe it is possible to reverse this damage to a large extent if less fatty food comes in and reduces the rate of storage. Diet doesn't matter as long as it's one that cuts calories and reduces fat and simple carbs. The researchers also noted that fish oil modulates some of the negative effects of fats and carbs.

They also caution that when people change their daily diets, they must be patient, because it takes time for the brain's metabolic messaging system to heal.

However, the research also indicated the researchers' beliefs that adding in short bursts of intermittent exercise throughout a day can be better than one single vigorous workout in terms of convincing your brain that you are full. This was offered as a result of a new study published in the *Journal of Obesity*. This study used blood testing every 15 minutes on participants who did no exercise on one day, 60 minutes of exercise on the next day, and on the third day twelve five-minute bouts of exercise. The blood tested the hormones related to the levels of hunger of the participants. On the second day, their hormone levels were the same but on the third day when they did shorter bursts of exercise throughout the day, they felt 32% fuller between 1:00 and 3:00 and between 3:00 and 5:00. The researchers concluded that staying physically active with brisk five-minute walks or other exercise throughout the day is essential to keeping hunger levels low.

Which is Best for Weight Loss? Aerobic or Resistance Training, or a Combination of Both?

A recent study at Duke University Medical Center was performed with overweight participants who were not doing exercise before the study. They were divided into three groups: an aerobics group worked out on treadmills, elliptical or cyclergometers to 75-80% of their maximum heart rate, which is considered vigorous aerobic exercise, for 45 minutes, three days a week, for over eight months. A second group did resistance training of three sets of 8 - 12 reps on eight resistance machines for major muscle groups, three days a week. The third group did everything both groups did.

Both the aerobics participants and the combination group lost weight while the resistance group gained weight due to building lean body mass.

Fat mass and waist circumference declined in the aerobics and combination groups, but there was no change in the resistance group.

The researchers, however, do recommend resistance training as very important to people ages 50-60 and older. This demographic naturally does lose muscle mass, which limits their physical functions in general.

High Intensity Interval Training

High Intensity Interval Training (HIIT) is an aerobic program of short bursts of energy to the point of exhaustion followed by a period of active rest such as light jogging.

The Department of Health recommends moderate aerobic activity 150 minutes a week, or 75 minutes a week of vigorous exercising. Sessions should be at least 10 minutes.

A recent study on the Hadza people on their metabolic rate, exercise intensity levels, and weight loss showed that if diet increases - calorie consumption along with increased exercise and intensity level - there will still be weight gain with increased calorie consumption. The study indicated that metabolism is not greatly affected by exercise alone, but that diet must be monitored along with an exercise program to reach the weight loss goals intended.

The News on Short Bursts of Cardio

Recently, many participants and followers of HIIT, for weight and fat loss, point to the value of short burst cardio activities for better results, compared to long and slow cardio workouts.

According to medical professionals reporting in the *Journal Of Obesity*, moving limbs very fast generates high levels of hormones called catecholamine, which are involved in the release of stored fat, notably abdominal and visceral fat, to be burned by the working muscles. Also, sprinting for 8 seconds raises the heart rate while keeping lactic acid release with normally tense muscles to a minimum. The workout is a very short duration - just 20 minutes of an alternating 8 seconds of hard level aerobics with 12 seconds of easy level aerobics for a total of 60 sprints.

The idea of a lesser amount of time spent on a more effective exercise is a great motivating factor health professionals agree on.

Moving Forward

Everyone is looking for that magic weight loss plan that will help you lose weight "without working out." Stop wishing and waiting, because the truth is, that is just NEVER going to happen. But you CAN get in shape and get healthy "without exercise" if you stop thinking about moving, using energy, having fun, and being active, as "exercise" and consider it a part of your healthy lifestyle.

10
KEEPING IT OFF AND STAYING HEALTHY

"Wow, what an accomplishment!"

That's the truth, whether you are just beginning your journey to a more fulfilling life, are somewhere along your pathway, or you've just beaten your previous best on a completed goal.

But getting there is only half the battle - now you have to stay there, and that means maintenance. Fear not, you got this far and you have your new-found knowledge and foresight and proven methods to guarantee that your body has the best chance possible for optimal health, being vigorous, gung-ho, fighting disease and infection, providing for long life, repairing the body as it needs - and you feel and look better than ever before.

What is most important is that you feel satisfied in your daily life with your eating and activities. These are true pleasures of life. And when you find your best path, and achieve your goals, you have made an amazing lifestyle change. You deserve to "keep on keeping on" for the best healthy you.

Mainstays of Maintenance

A recent study reported in the *American Journal of Preventive Medicine* documented 18 different practices of individuals that were associated with successful weight loss. The study also found that there were different methods that contributed to successfully keeping it off. The top three practices for successful weight loss maintenance were described by the following groups of dieters:

1. Those who reported limiting the amount of carbs they ate were 2.38 times more likely to report success with weight loss maintenance.

2. Those who reported following a consistent exercise routine were 2.94 times more successful at weight loss maintenance.

3. Those who reported eating plenty of low fat protein were 2.50 times more successful at weight loss maintenance.

In addition to these three top best practices for weight loss maintenance, this study and other studies related the following practices to successful weight loss maintenance:

Strategies of weighing oneself, planning meals, tracking fat and calories, exercising at least 30 minutes daily and adding physical activity into a daily life's routine scheduling.

The level of dietary restraint the individual mastered. Before weight loss a lower level ability to restrain uncontrolled and emotional eating and recognizing how to restrain oneself from binge eating had less weight loss and abilities to maintain weight loss, while those who were able to establish better restraint behaviors that decreased hunger and binging had large weight losses and greater successes in maintenance.

Monthly contact with an educator, or a physician even briefly, was shown to be more effective in maintaining weight loss than other interactive means such as web. It was noted that doctors can reinforce healthy habits, monitor weight and BMI and measurements, and even encourage further counseling and support.

People who had good levels of social support and strategies for dealing with any eating and exercising challenges, as well as abilities and strategies for dealing with life stress, recognizing and ability to shoulder life's responsibilities showed better weight loss maintenance results.

On the other side, *The American Journal of Preventive Medicine* study, as well as studies by the National Weight Control Registry, revealed factors that most predicted regaining weight loss.

These factors are:

- Believing that you are too tired to exercise
- Believing you have no time to exercise
- Believing it is too hard to keep an exercise or activity routine going
- Lack of social support to encourage diet plans and exercise

More uncontrolled eating, binging, intense hunger strikes, continuance of eating because of stress and emotions, inactive problem solving and shouldering of responsibilities showed great risk of weight regain.

Strong motivation to lose weight, feelings of confidence that one would achieve success, and feelings that he or she is autonomous in the decisions for weight loss, exercise, and life style choices had good indications for successful weight loss maintenance.

The National Weight Control Registry reported that those members successful in losing weight and maintaining the loss showed these top means:

- 78% ate breakfast daily
- 75% weigh themselves once a week
- 62% watch less than 10 hours of TV a week
- 90% exercise an average of 1 hour a day
- Participants limit the number of times they eat out to three times a week and eat fast food less than once a week
- They don't splurge too much on holidays
- They eat similar foods regularly

All of the participants who lost at least 30 pounds or more and maintained the loss for at least one year or longer used both diet and exercise to both lose the weight, and to maintain the weight loss.

Many other scientifically based studies corroborate the NWCR findings on diet and exercise for successful weight loss maintenance. All show that these strategies are important: weighing oneself, planning meals, tracking fat and calories, exercising at least 30 minutes a day, adding physical activity into a daily routine, reducing amounts of fast foods eaten, rewarding yourself for sticking to your life plans with diet and exercise, reminding yourself of your reasons why weight control is important to you.

Finally, another interesting study showed that for those with spouses who either are or are not on a weight loss/weight maintenance goals and plan, having open lines of communication relating to body image, acceptance, and the type of food that is shared could impact weight loss. If your spouse loses weight, it's been shown to positively affect you to lose weight and maintain the loss. The research explains that both weight gain and weight loss are contagious, affecting other members of the same family.

Your Kitchen and Home

You probably have already made changes to your household food items, shopping lists, and eating habits. But make sure your kitchen is always stocked with enough proper pans to prepare all varieties of health foods.

You should have a grill pan, steamer, zip-lock bags and storage containers to create fresh, healthy meals and freeze left-overs for later lunches or snacks. You should also have measuring cups and a food scale for accurate portion control.

Look at print and online magazines for healthy alternative recipes to add to your favorites - they can often give you inspiration to try new foods with their gorgeous photos and new ideas.

Keep the junk foods purged.

Keep a stock of healthy basics such as cans of tuna, salmon, sardines, chick peas, canned or frozen veggies, seasonings, vinegars, mustards, lemons and limes, tomato sauce, low sodium soy sauce, frozen unsweetened fruit, and Greek yogurts.

Keep up with your reward system. You always deserve a pat on the back in your own appreciative way for making daily healthy choices.

Minding Your Mindfulness

When you are fully present in the moment and not judging yourself, you hear your body cues loud and clear, you break free from your inner doubts and are really in the present enjoying each moment. Keep it going with your eating and your activity and exercise.

Avoid These Pitfalls:

Comparing yourself to others often leads to finding yourself drenched in extra deep puddles of self doubt, self criticism, self consciousness and those things can get you off your healthy course. A little comparison is, of course, normal for everyone, but notice it when it arises and starts to bog you down.

Shopping. Never shop when you are hungry. Always have a healthy snack before shopping.

Don't feel embarrassed to ask friends who invite you to dinner to please plan their entertaining with some lower fat, healthy foods, and then give them some clear cut suggestions.

When out socializing with friends or family, it's OK for you to suggest places with healthy alternatives on the menu that match your new lifestyle. Check websites to find places that have choices you, and your companions can both enjoy.

Remember to enjoy your life. Have fun, make sure that diet and exercise do not take over your life but becomes one of the many enjoyable parts.

Hungry? Grab a quick glass of water or flavored seltzer, or if you're still hungry after that, have one of your healthy snacks you have available.

Get Enough Sleep. The past president of the Obesity Society summarized numerous studies which show that with more sleep, individuals have a greater sense of fullness because sleep deprivation upsets the hormonal balance and triggers leptin which helps you feel full. Too little sleep triggers ghrelin, which in turn triggers hunger.

The key is moderation rather than deprivation. Eat well and exercise in a way that you can live with.

Mind Over Fatter

The term "physical fitness" causes a lot of confusion for people, and may be why they fail in their attempts to get in shape. It is because they place too much emphasis on the "physical" part. Health and fitness pros know that the path to true health and wellness can only be accomplished by taking an overall mind-body-sprit approach to "physical fitness."

By redefining the ways you look at diet and exercise, not so much as a way to "build muscle," or to "lose weight," but as a way to get your mind and body working together to reduce stress and to achieve peak performance, the more likely you will be to reach your fitness goals…whatever they may be.

REFERENCES

http://www.cdc.gov/nchs/fastats/overwt.htm

http://fit.webmd.com/kids/food/article/mindful-eating

http://www.health.harvard.edu/newsletters/Harvard_Mental_Health_Letter/2012/February/why-stress-causes-people-to-overeat

http://www.mayoclinic.com/health/weight-loss/NU00616/NSECTIONGROUP=2
http://www.oprah.com/health/Americas-Next-Great-Diet-Craze#ixzz2dZFlYZ4h

http://www.oprah.com/health/Americas-Next-Great-Diet-Craze/2#ixzz2dZFznmev

http://www.oprah.com/health/Americas-Next-Great-Diet-Craze/3#ixzz2dZG6sebf

http://www.foxnews.com/health/2013/06/13/new-diet-craze-offers-five-days-feasting-for-two-days-famine/#ixzz2dZGWXemf

http://www.aafp.org/afp/2010/0915/p630.html

http://www.scientificamerican.com/article.cfm?id=control-your-urges-with-a-ride-on-the-mindbus&WT.mc_id=SA_syn

http://www.ajpmonline.org/article/S0749-3797(10)00474-5/abstract

http://yourlife.usatoday.com/fitness-food/weight-loss-challenge/story/2011-10-12/Analysis-finds-it-is-possible-to-maintain-weight-loss/50745306/1

http://www.hindawi.com/journals/jobes/2012/480467/

http://www.nydailynews.com/life-style/health/diet-trump-exercise-weight-loss-article-1.1430729#ixzz2gebwEK9g

http://gma.yahoo.com/armless-body-builder-inspires-fitness-world-her-ability-101506751--abc-news-health.html

http://www.whfoods.com/nutrientstoc.php

http://www.caloriecontrol.org/articles-and-video/feature-articles/study-identifies-foods-that-promote-weight-maintenance

http://www.motleyhealth.com/weight-loss/four-steps-to-a-healthy-weight#ixzz2e0mxHlaT

http://www.diabetes.org/food-and-fitness/fitness/weight-loss/setting-realistic-weight-loss.html

http://www.diabetes.org/food-and-fitness/fitness/weight-loss/weight-loss-matters-tip.html

http://health.howstuffworks.com/wellness/diet-fitness/weight-loss/how-to-start-a-weight-loss-pogram.html

http://healthland.time.com/2012/07/13/the-secrets-to-weight-loss-keep-a-food-journal-dont-skip-meals-eat-in/#ixzz2e119wsec

http://healthland.time.com/2012/07/13/the-secrets-to-weight-loss-keep-a-food-journal-dont-skip-meals-eat-in/#ixzz2e11P8PoC

Deepening the measurement of motivation in the physical activity domain: Introducing behavioural resolve, Psychology of Sport and Exercise, Volume 14, Issue 4, July 2013, Pages 455-460 Ryan E. Rhodes, Lori Horne

http://www.caloriecontrol.org/articles-and-video/feature-articles/study-identifies-foods-that-promote-weight-maintenance

Building a Practically Useful Theory of Goal Setting and Task Motivation, Edwin A. Locke, Gary P. Latham, American Psychology 2002;57:705-17

http://www.centerformedicalweightloss.com/blog/2013/02/25/goal-setting-can-you-reach-too-high/

http://www.prweb.com/releases/2013/7/prweb10920532.htmhttp://selfregulationlab.nl/wp-content/uploads/2013/05/De-Vet-et-al-2013-J-Health-Psychol.pdf

http://www.dailymail.co.uk/health/article-2134162/Research-shows-trying-lose-weight-alters-brain-hormones-youre-doomed-pile-again.html#ixzz2dYTL83VP

http://www.rd.com/health/diet-weight-loss/13-things-you-never-knew-about-your-weight/#ixzz2dYUYB4SF8.

http://www.rd.com/health/diet-weight-loss/13-things-you-never-knew-about-your-weight/#ixzz2dYUioeWI

http://abcnews.go.com/Health/100-million-dieters-20-billion-weight-loss-industry/story?id=16297197

http://www.gallup.com/poll/150986/lose-weight-americans-rely-dieting-exercise.aspx

http://www.ncbi.nlm.nih.gov/pubmed/22681398 Why do individuals not lose more weight from an exercise intervention at a defined dose? An energy balance analysis. Thomas DM, Bouchard C, Church T, Slentz C, Kraus WE, Redman LM, Martin CK, Silva AM, Vossen M, Westerterp K, Heymsfield SB. Center for Quantitative Obesity Research, Montclair State University, Montclair, NJ 07043, USA. © 2012 The Authors. obesity reviews © 2012 International Association for the Study of Obesity. PMID: 22681398 [PubMed - indexed for MEDLINE]

http://womensrunning.competitor.com/2013/03/health-wellness/why-you-cant-lose-weight_11491

http://signup.weightwatchers.com/util/art/archive.aspx?tabnum=3&sc=802

http://prowellness.vmhost.psu.edu/wp-content/uploads/weight_loss_weight-lossMaint_PRO-Wellness.pdf

http://www.medscape.com/viewarticle/555511

http://www.news-medical.net/news/20110705/Practices-associated-with-successful-weight-loss-versus-maintenance.aspx

http://dx.doi.org/10.5402/2013/395125 Body Weight Perception and Weight Control Practices among Teenagers

http://www.choosemyplate.gov/food-groups/

http://www.nutrition.gov/weight-management

The National Weight Control Registry. See "Long-term Weight Maintenance" in American Journal of Clinical Nutrition, Vol. 82, No. 1, 222S-225S, July 2005

www.supertracker.usda.gov/default.aspx

http://www.choosemyplate.gov/ http://www.choosemyplate.gov/food-groups/physicalactivity_calories_used_table.html cjhart

Methods for Voluntary Weight Loss and Control. National Institutes of Health Technology Assessment Conference. Annals of Internal Medicine. 119(7, Part 2), October 1, 1993.

Choosing a Safe and Successful Weight-Loss Program, U.S. Department of Health and Human Services, Public Health Service, National Institutes of Health, National Institute of Diabetes & Digestive & Kidney Diseases, NIH Publication No. 08-3700, April 2008. http://www.win.niddk.nih.gov/publications/choosing.html

http://www.health.gov/DietaryGuidelines

http://www.consumer.ftc.gov/topics/health-fitness

http://www.consumer.ftc.gov/articles/0061-weighing-claims-diet-ads

http://www.nutrition.gov/weight-management/what-you-should-know-about-popular-diets

http://www.fda.gov/Food/IngredientsPackagingLabeling/LabelingNutrition/ucm274593.htm

http://www.cdc.gov/physicalactivity/growingstronger/motivation/define.html

http:/www.marinpsychologist.blogspot.com

http://www.marksdailyapple.com/10-psychological-hurdles-keeping-you-from-losing-weight-and-how-to-overcome-them/#ixzz2dSh328RO

http://www.cfah.org/hbns/2011/losing-weight-keeping-it-off-might-require-distinct-skill-sets#.UiCvL-bD-00 Out To Lunch July 5, 2011

ABOUT THE AUTHOR

Greg Justice is an international best-selling author, speaker, and fitness entrepreneur. He opened AYC Health & Fitness, Kansas City's original personal training center, in May 1986, and has personally trained more than 48,000 one-on-one sessions. Today, AYC specializes in corporate wellness, group fitness, and personal training.

He has been actively involved in the fitness industry for more than three decades as a club manager, owner, personal fitness trainer, and corporate wellness supervisor. Greg currently serves on the advisory board of two personal training schools. He mentors and instructs trainers worldwide through his coaching programs and Corporate Boot Camp System class.

Greg writes articles for many publications and websites, is a featured columnist for *Corporate Wellness Magazine*, and his monthly column, "Treadmill Talk," is published in *Personal Fitness Professional* magazine. He is the author of five books including *Mind Your Own Fitness, A Mindful Approach To Exercise, Lies & Myths About Corporate Wellness*, and *Treadside Manner, Confessions Of A Serial Personal Trainer*.

Greg holds a master's degree in HPER (exercise science) and a bachelor's degree in Health & Physical Education from Morehead State University, Morehead, KY.

Made in the USA
Charleston, SC
11 April 2014